Striving

for

Imprefection

per

SCOTT "Q" MARCUS

THINspirational Columnist and Recovering Perfectionist

Another year's worth of
^52 Inspirational
Playful Columns
on Living Well,
Changing Habits,
and Other Acts of Faith

Striving for Imperfection
Volume 5

ISBN: 978-1466436176

Printed in the United States of America

For additional copies of this book, or to hire Scott "Q" Marcus for
speaking, coaching, workshops, or consulting, please call 707.442.6243 or
scottq@scottqmarcus.com.

To get past what holds you — or your business — back,
go to www.ThisTimeIMeanIt.com
or
or www.ScottQMarcus.com

To my readers, without whom none of these volumes would be possible.

TABLE OF CONTENTS

Striving

for

Imprefection

per

Scott "Q" Marcus

THINspirational Columnist and Recovering Perfectionist

Another year's worth of
^52 Inspirational
Playful Columns
on Living Well,
Changing Habits,
and Other Acts of Faith

THE ONLY RESOLUTION THAT WORKS

STOP! DON'T DO IT! I know it's the "new year," that ritualistic period whereby we become fixated on ridding ourselves of that sluggish, bloated, overloaded blob-like feeling in which we wrapped ourselves for the previous two months. Whipped up by cartons of cookies and bags of breadstuffs; flavored by truckloads of turkey with gravy, ham with glaze, or both; coated in tankards of eggnog (with and without rum); we are just darn-near ready to put on the brakes and embrace our "new me."

It is a cultural happening. As ubiquitous was "Have a Holly Jolly Christmas" last month are now the signs of this new year's dawning. Full-page gift ads have converted to double truck spreads promoting six-pack abs and shriek, "Have the sexy glutes you've always wanted!" Even jolly old Saint Nick has shifted his routine. Two weeks ago, singing elves warmly patted their bellies after consuming plates of iced cookies. Today? Santa's helpers wear sweatpants and can barely let forth a hum as they aspire to get heart rates into the target zone while pounding away on the treadmill in the new North Pole gym.

Our entire national psyche has clunked over from, "how much can I eat?" to "Oh my goodness! How will I undo what I have done?" We are ready – daresay eager – to toss away yesterday's consume-all mentality in the same fashion as we pitched torn wrapping paper into the recycling bin not very long ago.

Hmmm...maybe recycling bin is a bad analogy. After all, that means it will be reused. Or – on second thought – maybe it's accurate. After all, how many times have we traveled this same tattered, threadbare, circular path? One might say we don't throw away our habits; we merely recycle them. I applaud the concept, "Renew, reuse, recycle." However, in this instance, it might be better to stop with "Renew."

Nothing changes if nothing changes.

To merely raise your right hand and solemnly spout forth, "This year, I will..." does not guarantee next year will begin differently than did this one. The primary cause of the yearly February condition known as "RF" (Resolution Fatigue) is a misunderstanding of how to accomplish our objectives. Many think that the key is to dream bigger, reach further, aim higher. They also might think french fries come from France. (They'd be wrong on both accounts.)

We do that because we so want our results NOW! We want to be "there" as soon as possible. But, no matter how hard we stomp our feet, and cry "foul," change does not work that way. Change does not – poof – happen! Rather, it evolves. Sometimes it inches forward, oft times it slides backwards. Like life, it does not travel a straight path. As example, if I desire to lose 30 pounds, I cannot put together a plan for the endpoint. Instead I must first learn how to drop one and actually keep it off. Small goal – repeat as necessary.

Resolutions, goals, promises – whatever we might label them – collapse because we target the broad goal rather than shoot for small long-lasting changes.

Want to know the only resolution that works? Give up on yearly resolutions. Make them small. Make them often, and make sure they stick. Everything else will take care of itself.

THE ROPE

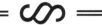

When I was in school, it was uncool to admit it. Things change, thank God. Therefore, let me push my glasses up on my nose, put my pens in my pocket protector, adjust my suspenders, and proudly announce, "I am a science geek!" I feel better now, thank you for listening.

My biggest regrets (so far) are that I will never achieve Warp Factor Nine sitting next to Number One on the Starship Enterprise, nor sail the dark reaches of space with Commander Adama. I hope for someone like Neo to come forth and rescue me from the insanity that sometimes seems to surround us, and – especially on rough days – can accept that we are indeed deep within the Matrix.

When bored, and being said "science geek," I will sometimes engage in "thought experiments," imagined scenarios attempting to explain certain real-world effects or at times used to enhance creativity.

As illustration, imagine a very long pulley system where the cord reaches from your front yard all the way around the moon and back to where you stand. At the terminus is fastened a weight. Now, suppose you tugged on the front end of the rope, what would happen to the weight on the other end?

At first blush, the answer appears obvious, "Well, of course, it would rise." After all, that's how pulley's work, pull one side, the other responds.

"A-ha! Gotcha!" Nothing travels faster than light, which requires almost three seconds to travel the distance from the Earth to the Moon and back. Therefore, even in the fastest scenario, it would take at least that long for the weight to lift. Otherwise the rope would have traveled faster than light, which is impossible. Yet the force used to yank on the rope had to have some effect, to go somewhere didn't it? What happened to it?

Want to know the answer? Actually, so would I; there isn't one. Like I said, it's a thought experiment. Its purpose is to cause you to think.

"Well, that's all fine and dandy Scott," you say; "But if I wanted experiments, I'd buy a chemistry set. What does that have to do with anything?"

I'm glad you asked.

Every January, we have an almost cultural knee-jerk reflex: start imagining how the year will end, and where will we be? What would we like to achieve personally and professionally? How much money would we like to earn – and what will we do with it when we do? What about health; lose weight, gain weight, be more active, stop smoking? So many questions, so many opportunities, unlimited possibilities; all await our choices. So, we devise plans, we establish goals, dare I say it – we make resolutions. Our intentions are laudable but so often are actions are lamentable.

Why?

We rarely attempt today what could possibly be delayed. "There's always tomorrow," we say, "What's the rush? I have plenty of time."

There might be "plenty of time," we never know; moreover that is

At home, our damage was limited to several dishes and picture frames, as well as the several hours necessary to reassemble our lives. Everything is now back in its place, where it will remain – until the next quake.

We have been sent a reminder. Although a few people were injured and there was severe property damage, there was not one fatality and very few serious injuries.

As a community, we will rebuild, helping each other, letting our differences be put aside in the interest of the greater good and a common humanity that we many time forget. By reaching out and pulling others closer, we become stronger, and create a better, healthier community for all of us.

We are so fortunate; sometimes we need a reminder.

LESSON LEARNED

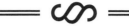

OK class, today's assignment is to create the most annoying place ever; ready?

Let's begin by populating it with lots of tired, irritable inhabitants confined to a cramped area with hardly any places to rest and absolutely no spot to get comfortable. Many of these folks will wear too much perfume or, better yet, haven't seen the working end of a shower in days. Of course, the whole environment has to be far from home, and – oh yes – let's make it extremely loud.

Now, let's spruce up the annoyance factor by tossing in some arcane commands.

Rule one: You are only allowed to have in your ownership one container of essential items; but the consequences for possessing those is that is you must drag them behind you wherever you go; a ball and chain. Rule Two: Not for a minute can you let them leave your custody. If you want to add more items, you can purchase from a very limited supply of things that will be far more costly than they should be, and you must stand in long lines to obtain them (don't forget, you must have your container always in tow). Rule Three: Nosy, ill-mannered, discourteous natives will handle and interrogate you at will, sporadically rummage through your package of personal belongings, and time after time subject you to yet additional seemingly useless rules which may change at any time.

I think we're done. What shall we call it? Dante's Inferno? Hell? How about, "An Airport?"

Traveling has a knack to make anybody cranky; so, I had empathy for the nine-year-old with the pink suitcase waiting in the petrified line to board the jet. Her dad, bent close to her, staring unflinchingly into her eyes, was wagging his finger for emphasis and scolding her sotto voce. "We don't push people out of the way. We wait our turn, do you understand?"

Her eyes drilling into the floor of the gateway, an angry expression contorting her face, she rocked defiantly from side-to-side, holding steadfast, "He's not 'people;' he's my little brother! And he's slow! I want to get on the airplane all ready! I'm tired!"

"I understand," replied her father, "We're all frustrated. But that doesn't excuse pushing. Are we clear?"

"I want to get on the airplane!" She stomped her foot for emphasis and crossed her arms across her chest.

"We will go on the airplane when you apologize to Robbie. Tell him you're sorry."

Begrudgingly realizing she had no choice and finally accepting the parameters, she faced her sibling, mumbled something, then looked back at Dad.

"Very good," he said; hugged her, rose to his full height and took her by the hand as the family proceeded forward. She had learned her lesson, her reward being that she now able to proceed to her objective.

As I watched the drama, it dawned on me that this process does not end when we move away from our parents. It is a sequence that presents itself continually: Frustration. Lesson. Acceptance. Progress. Repeat cycle as necessary until learned.

The only difference between those of us with single-digit ages and smooth skin, and those of us with a few years under our belts and a road map of wrinkles, is that we aren't always fortunate enough to have someone explain the guidelines so clearly.

FEBRUARY RESOLUTIONS

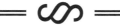

One can always tell the time of year by the dominant color at the greeting card stores. Starting with Spring, we begin the pastel season. We advance without delay into the "red, white, and blue" period; followed by "Orange and Black;" with a brief flurry of "Brown, Red, Orange and Forest Green" in November. (The colors for the latter part of the year shift quickly because the "Red Green" season dominates everything.) We conclude this colorful journey with the "RED! RED! RED!" season, a period into which we are now firmly ensconced.

Aside from romance, this time of year also sadly signifies a type of break up; the ending of well-intentioned resolutions proudly and honorably stated just four short weeks ago.

I have never been a big fan of resolutions. I've never done them; I don't think I ever will. Don't get me wrong; I absolutely firmly believe that making commitments and setting goals are essential if I want to direct the changes in my life. I also don't have a problem in the world with making them in January. I mean, sure, why not? January's as good as any month.

But that's the point: January's as good as any month. Why do we feel that if we "blow it" in January, we can't reestablish them some other time? Why not put forth a "February commitment;" or honor the father of our country's honesty with a "George Washington Day

Promise;" or pick Valentine's Day to state my "love-myself-enough-to-change" vows? Granted, they might sound ridiculous; but are those dates of any less value than January 1?

Choosing goals basically because it's a "that time of year" (and that's when everybody does them) makes us less inclined to achieve them. Why? Because they're not driven by an inner aspiration, but rather forced by external dynamics.

Long-term change (does any other type matter?) must be borne from within, not pushed upon us by outside forces. Yes, external drivers, such as weighing a certain amount, not fitting into your clothes, crossing a landmark age, going through a break-up, or losing a job; can be powerful triggers. Each will get you moving, for sure. But, once the initial pain has diminished, so does the drive to continue the very behavior which caused its dissipation.

In order to beyond doubt achieve life-changing objectives, it is imperative that I do it for ME, not because it's a certain time of year, or my doctor said to, or because everyone thinks I should. I must move forward because it truly matters to me in my core. In other words, I do it because I want the results of my efforts, not because I am told to change.

So, if you're finding that flame of January has faded cold chunk of coal today, and you wish to move forward, ask yourself three questions:

- "What's ONE cool thing I will get from this effort?" We usually give up not because we don't want our goals, but because we lost sight of WHY we wanted them.

- Next, what's ONE small step that I'd actually do to achieve that benefit? Remember, small steps done regularly get better results than large one done intermittently

- Finally, will I do it TODAY? If your answer is "No," you've chosen the wrong goal. Be honest. Remember, goals are not to impress others; they're to benefit you. If you're not going to begin right now – for whatever reason – this is not your aspiration. Choose something else – which you can do any time of the year.

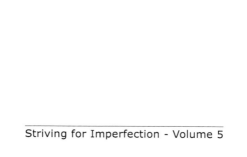

TEN YEARS AFTER

The last thing we did together was to watch the Nathan Lane/Robin Williams movie, "Birdcage," just the two of us alone at my aunt's house. My cousin had taken his mother to his place so my mom and I could spend an evening alone before I flew home the next day.

Ruth Marcus and Mildred Plotkin were two of three sisters, born in the twenties. Eleanor Diamond, the youngest member of the triad stayed in Michigan, but these two were within minutes of each other, so together they had driven the road of life for over 70 years. Through five births, one divorce, several deaths, three bar mitzvahs, one bat mitzvah, eight weddings of their children (including second marriages), and countless holidays filled with matzo ball soup and tasteless chicken; they supported each other during the difficult times and celebrated during joyful ones. They could – in one moment – drive each other crazy, and within seconds defend each other against overwhelming odds.

"No one – NO ONE – messes with our family!" My mom emphatically reminded me many times, usually when she felt someone was taking advantage of me. Although basically peaceful, she was a tigress if she felt her family was being mistreated.

The time had now arrived for these two sisters to take together one last ride. Aunt Millie would be with her to the end. However, she was no spring chicken and needed to build up some strength for the upcoming trip. My presence in town allowed her at least for a night that freedom.

"How are you feeling, mom?" I asked.

Sitting in the rocker, cradling a cup of hot tea, a quilted blanket on her legs and several vials of pills on the table next to her, she replied, "I'm still fine honey. You don't need to ask me every few minutes. I promise to tell you if I need anything, all right?"

"Sure, Mom. I'm sorry. I just…" I just what? To be brutally honest, I was really anxious with the whole dying thing and checking in with her helped reassure me. I had never been in this position and felt woefully out of anything that might have even come close to a comfort zone.

Of course, my mother had never been in her position either. Yet, she accepted it with grace. As if reading my mind, she said, "You know sweetie, in some ways, it's kind of exciting. I don't want to go; but I am curious. It's my last journey. Who knows what I'll learn?"

Pause. No reply from me.

Softly, "I'm okay Scott. I really am. Don't worry."

I stopped staring at my shoes and looked up. There she was, smiling through me with her trademarked piercing, I'm-proud-of-you-even-if-you-don't-know-what-to-do gaze; more concerned for me than for herself.

"Mom, can you stop staring? It's making me uncomfortable."

"I just want to soak you in."

"I know. But can you soak me in while we do something else at the same time?"

"Of course sweetie. Why don't we put on the movie?"

I pushed the play button and turned toward the screen. My mother continued drilling into my soul with her eyes.

"Aren't you going to watch?" I asked, trying to divert her attention.

"You watch. I'll soak."

February fifth marks ten years. Sometimes, I still feel her gaze. It doesn't bother me in the slightest; quite the contrary, I miss it more than I can say.

DEALING WITH STRESS

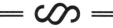

Sometimes, I tend to be an eensy-weensy bit resistant to changing how I act. The bottom line is that I, like most folks, really do like my habits. I complain about them and tell others I'll change (more to get them off my back than for anything else). I do recognize that they might not always be the healthiest patterns, but – you know – they're warm and cozy and make it so I don't have to think so much, which takes loads of energy. Therefore, it's easier to pour a glass of wine, put on reality TV, and turn away from my thoughts than it is to anxiously ruminate on everything requiring adjusting. Besides, I rationalize, there's always tomorrow, isn't there?

Yet, once in a while, something crashes through that dense wall of denial and I can no longer avoid looking.

Today, at a very powerful, presentation, I learned that the three leading causes of death in the U.S. in 1900 (Pneumonia, Influenza, and Tuberculosis) are not even in the top five 100 years later (heart disease, Cancer, and stroke). In effect, over the span of an extended lifetime, our biggest health concerns have shifted from being "attacked from the outside" to being "attacked from the inside." That's a powerful bit of data.

Part of the reason is that we are now under constant, unending, ongoing, chronic stress. Sure, we're not fighting off sabertooth tigers anymore; but we pay too many bills with too few dollars, or we attempt too many things with too little time, or both, or more. Our body can't perceive the difference between "sabertooth tiger stress" and the "IRS is on the phone for you" stress. All it understands is that something is a kilter; we are under pressure. (Whether the stress is caused by actual or perceived events makes no difference; we respond the same.)

Couple that fact with the detail that our modern diet is so out of whack that nutritionists refer to it as "hyper inflammatory." That means that when threatened, our body throws the preverbal kitchen sink at almost any problem. Instead of marshalling a couple of "antibiotic soldiers" to quell a minor disturbance, it delivers an entire, heavily-armed, fully equipped battalion. Once the threat has been eliminated, those extra soldiers hang around with nothing to do – except leave waste products. Blend that with our constant stress-level, and well, we've got bunkers of waste-producing soldiers camped out all over our insides, lining our cells with all sorts of unnecessary non-disposable nasties.

Since stress is beyond our control, we cannot dispel it and send the soldiers on leave. Rather, we can only disarm the situation by thinking differently, moving more, and changing how we eat.

Here's where today's talk made its impact on me. Eric, the presenter, offered clear, easy-to-implement ideas to begin to reverse the course. Take some Fish Oil, increase Vitamin D, drink Green Tea now and then. He was honest; it's not a panacea; it's merely a few doable actions that can improve one's heath. They are things I can do right now – and I did.

Not only are simple ideas usually the best, but, now knowing what I've learned, they don't stress me out as much as doing nothing.

It's not that difficult

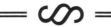

Sometimes – one might even argue "always" – wisdom and truth are found in the most basic statements. One of the simplest, yet most empowering comments I have heard is from Dr. Sue Morter. Aside from being a powerhouse speaker, she's extremely inspirational, a dynamo on the stage, and outstandingly wise.

"So, what did liberating life-altering observation did she lay pass unto you?" You ask, breathless with anticipation.

"It's difficult until it isn't."

"Huh? That's it?"

Yep; five words; seven if you don't count contractions. But, consider the message in that unvarnished declaration. Most of what we want for ourselves is really not difficult to obtain. We possess the tools (or know where to get them) and we know what we desire; all we have to do is go get it. The hitch in the giddy up is how we assemble the plan, making it complex and complicated. We smother it with all makeup of parameters to which we really cannot – or do not want to – abide. We spend so much energy building the golden pathway that we're too exhausted to walk upon it.

As case in point, how 'bout we look at losing weight? (Wow, who would think I'd choose that as an example?) The bottom line of weight loss is brilliantly clear: Eat less; move more. Period. No pills, no programs, no late-night TV promises. See? That's not difficult, is it? If I regularly shut my mouth a few minutes earlier and move my feet a couple of steps further, the pounds "magically" falls away. We all know that. Yet, because we're in such a hurry to "get there," we go overboard in the implementation and develop barriers to actually achieving what we want.

Boldly, I stand tall, placing my fists upon my hips, puffing out my chest, and proclaiming to anyone who cares (and many who don't). "I am now on a diet! (Insert trumpets...) Therefore, until I lose 30 pounds, I shall not be able to go with my friends, family, or business associates to any eating establishment. While imprisoned in my barren, spartan, kitchen, I will consume only unprocessed, all-natural, organic, high-fiber, sugar-free, mostly tasteless, foodstuffs. Furthermore, I will rise two hours earlier each and every day and spend that time meditating, journaling, and exercising. I have calculated that this plan will shall allow me to lose three pounds a week, which I will do this day forth until I have achieved my goals." After my pronouncement, I twirl spectacularly on my heels, place nose firmly in the air and stomp dramatically into my self-established sensory-deprivation chamber, where I shall remain in exclusion until I have achieved a smaller waistline.

Hey Tinkerbell, can we put down the fairy-wand and step out from fantasyland for a moment?

What began as extremely unfussy and obtainable intention – eating better and moving more – has erupted into a full-scale mega-production requiring learning how to cook differently, shopping with new eyes, rearranging schedules, altering relationships, and devising self-inflicting intimidating goals. Building such blockades makes the procedure ridiculously difficult and horribly unpleasant.

After ramming one's head against the wall enough, we will look for doors, finally "letting go" and releasing as unproductive the artificial rules and limiting beliefs; which allows us to get down to basics. We find something we will actually do and take one small, simple, easy, baby step; which we repeat until we get actually get what we want.

It was difficult. Then it wasn't. It is up to each of us to determine when we want that to change.

Taking Responsibility

One of my best friends recently came home from a self-help seminar with that Oh-my-God-I've-just-experienced-a-life-changing-event kind of glow. One reason was *The Art of Possibility* by Rosamund Stone Zander and her husband, Boston Philharmonic Conductor Benjamin Zander. She was so blown away by the content of this manuscript that she bought every used copy she could find and asked – no, insisted – that her friends read it.

I always feel trepidation when a well-meaning person pushes a book into my hands. I know they want to share the good news with me; I appreciate the thoughtfulness. Moreover, it's not that I don't like reading; actually I do. It's just I wish I had more time to do so. I love sitting on the couch on a lazy, rainy, windy afternoon, wrapped in one of those blankets with sleeves, (diet) hot chocolate on the end table; lost in a brilliant yarn. Yet, my reality is that after a 60-hour week writing, researching, and preparing presentations; as well as following world events via web, magazine, and newsprint; would you think less of me when I admit that the only reading I end up doing with regularity is the programming guide the DVR splashes on the TV screen?

So when she planted the book in my hands and emphatically told me she really wanted to know what I thought, I felt trapped.

I'm glad I was.

The authors posit several "practices." They don't tell you how to use them, simply that they exist. The choice to utilize them – or not – is ours. Practices include: Be a Contributor, Light a Spark, and Give in to Passion, all wonderfully valid. However, the practice that prompted me to take keyboard to word processor is "Be the Board;" in effect, take responsibility for EVERYTHING that happens in your life, even if it doesn't seem like it was caused by you.

It's easy to take responsibility when it's something we do (OK, maybe it's not exactly "easy," but good people do it anyway). My interpretation of "Be the Board" is that we also must assume accountability for those things we did not do, as we are the board on which all our life's actions are played out. The pieces in that game are all connected to us, like it or not.

As example, should my marriage be in jeopardy because my spouse is uncaring and emotionally absent, a standard – arguably fair – reaction would be to blame her for my lousy marriage and feel miserable and trapped because of her. However, if I take responsibility for the situation in which I now find myself, I rapidly notice options I might not have seen otherwise. If I am trying to lose weight and, despite valiant, sincere, efforts, the scale does not move, standard modus operandi is to curse the diet and feel defeated. Taking responsibility however causes me to examine if there might be actions I could do I had not thought of before. This practice is equally powerful in professional or personal situations, and it begins with a simple change of thought.

Responsibility is not blame. Indeed it might *not* be my fault that I have trouble losing weight or choosing a good spouse, but it is my responsibility to change it if I wish to improve. After all, the word itself means "ability to respond." Without it, I am trapped, stagnant, petrified. Once I embrace my responsibility to improve my lot in life, I am empowered with unlimited options.

Weighing in on childhood obesity

Michelle Obama has chosen to grapple with the crisis of childhood obesity. Props to the First Lady, as this is a dilemma of historic proportion. In a mere two decades, when we as elderly baby boomers, are gobbling up every available resource related to health care, our children and grandchildren, plagued by the ailments of a lifetime of obesity, will figuratively be feeding from the same trough. (Bad analogy; but it works.) We are rapidly approaching the only time in history when three generations will be suffering from the ill effects of poor health at the same moment.

So, let me make one thing clear: childhood obesity begins in adulthood.

At first blush, that makes as much sense as the bumper sticker that proclaims, "Insanity is hereditary. You get it from your kids." Of course, that placard is humorous; the wellbeing of society is anything but. The unvarnished truth is when we get down to brass tacks, children to not become obese by choice, but rather by the (in) action of adults.

Before, with great high dudgeon, mothers and fathers converge upon this establishment carrying pitchforks and hoisting torches shouting for my removal, let me add with great haste (spoken as a father as well as a formerly obese child), that I am not placing fault entirely on the parents. Oh, indeed, there is blame to spread far and wide. However, we are the primary and first decision makers for our children. We set them on their path. We instill upon them our moral guidelines. We are the where the buck – or cookie – stops.

I know that in today's two-working-parent-I-am-really-exhausted-at-the-end-of-the-day world, fighting the influences heaped upon our offspring is overwhelming. I grok that these influences are powerful, selfish, misguided, even mal-intended. Yet, I think that as a society, we stand in a circular firing squad aiming at those on either side; in effect – pardon the mixed metaphor – fiddling as an overweight Rome burns in its own deep fryer.

Parents place fault with the media for an endless wave of advertising aimed at those too young to discern accuracy from hype. The media passes it to the schools for poor meal choices and vending machines full of sugar. Our educational system holds responsible government for inadequate funding, forcing subsidized income provided by the vendors who place the goodies in the machines, who then shout, "lack of control" at the parents. Circle complete; nothing is accomplished.

We have seen the problem and it is all of us. Someone has got to do something; no longer can we wait for "the other guy." It therefore stands to reason that since my children are the most important people in my life, I am the end of their line. I must step forward first, figuratively and literally.

I resolve, that before I collapse on to the softness of the couch at the end of a long day, I will take a 10-minute walk with my kids, giving them the example of activity and the support of listening. I promise to not bring into our house any product whose label has as its primary ingredient, sugar (or any kind of "–ose"). I agree to eat a little less and pay attention a little more. In effect, I will stand taller, striving to be the example I want my children to become.

Role models are not without flaws; however, they take responsibility for them and continually attempt to improve. That's an objective good for children of any age, no matter how wrinkled they might be on the outside.

Learning from mistakes

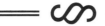

"Oops!"

"What do you mean, "oops"? Nothing good ever starts with 'oops.'"

"Really? I'm not sure about that. 'Oops' means I made a mistake."

"I know what it means; I'm not stupid. But it never leads anywhere good."

"I don't agree."

"OK, how 'bout this? I was at the dentist a few months ago. I was getting a tooth pulled…"

"Ouch; that's not fun."

"No, it's not. So, they've got me in that chair that looks like something from the Spanish Inquisition. My mouth is numb, I'm drooling like a one-year old – "

"Sounds attractive."

"Anyway… They have the chair leaning way back, the light is in my eyes, I've got one of those rubber things in my mouth – what do you call 'em?"

"Dental dam."

"Yeah, I've got a dental dam in my mouth and the dentist is yanking and pulling on my tooth. Suddenly the tooth pops loose, the dentist loses his grip, I hear him say, 'oops,' and before you know it, he's got me out of the chair, flipped over, patting me on the back like he's burping a baby."

"Wow! What happened?"

"Apparently, he dropped the tooth into my throat."

"Really? Was it dangerous?"

"Well, he was concerned that it could get in my lungs. But it didn't; apparently I swallowed it."

"So everything came out OK in the end?"

"Is that meant to be cute?"

"No, maybe I worded it poorly, but I meant what I said."

"Yeah, sure, I was fine."

"So 'oops' was a good thing then."

"No, it was a bad thing. He made a mistake. It could have had terrible results."

"But, it didn't, because he saw that he made a mistake, and corrected for it real quickly. Let's say, he didn't admit the mistake and just pretended that he still had your tooth in his pliers and just went about his business, not telling you what was going wrong."

"Well, that wouldn't have been smart. I could have got hurt."

"Right, because he admitted his mistake and he learned from it, things got better. And, you know what? I'll bet he's much more aware of that problem now then he was back then."

"I'm sure he is."

"So, future patients are probably better off, right?"

"Uh, yeah, I guess so."

"So admitting his mistake took care of you quickly and will help others prevent from experiencing what you experienced. That's two good things from one 'oops.'"

"But it's embarrassing to make mistakes."

"Maybe. But it's more embarrassing to make them repeatedly, isn't it?"

"Yes."

"So, the quicker we acknowledge we made a mistake and the sooner we adjust the better off we are."

"But, wouldn't it be better never to slip up?"

"Sure it would. And wouldn't the world be better if everything worked out exactly like we expect it to?"

"That's not going to happen."

"Spot on. And it's equally unrealistic to assume you won't screw-up now and then, especially if you're trying new things. So without mistakes, there is no reason for adjustment, which means we're not learning anything; therefore nothing changes. So, one could say mistakes are actually step one in improving our life."

"But only if we acknowledge them and change them."

"To do anything else would be a mistake."

IS YOUR DIET
MAKING YOU FAT?

The number one rule of the universe: "If I always do what I've always done, I'll always be where I've always been." Alas, despite the apparent (lack of) results of some dieting behaviors, we blindly pursue these non-starters.

Elisa Zied, RD, an American Dietetic Association spokesperson and author of "Feed Your Family Right!" listed five unproductive behaviors. I – always the helper – have added my own commentary.

Unproductive behavior #1: Saving your calories for dinner.

Although the unflinching truth is summed up as "calories in versus calories out," banking them for the end of the day apparently causes hunger hormones to go wild. (I'm picturing plump hormones partying on spring break in Florida – must delete mental image!)

Of course, this presupposes that those of us who trying to lose weight are actually paying attention to hunger, which we're not; we're on autopilot, shoveling greasy, gooey, syrupy goodness down our gullet without regard to taste nor need. If we were actually responding to hunger, we'd stop well before dinner anyway.

Behavior #2: "Grazing" instead of eating regularly scheduled meals.

I wasn't aware of this little tidbit, but women who eat regular meals burn more calories in the three hours after eating than those who unplanned meals. Sit down. Use a plate. Lose weight.

#3. Quick, crash diets to "look good" for a certain event.

Drastically cutting calories causes a loss of muscle with the fat – especially if you haven't been exercising. Muscle is one of the more important components of metabolism. High metabolism contributes to weight loss, while low metabolism causes one to be tired (and plump). The solution? Simply eat a little less than you want, and stay with that for a while. Besides, let's be honest, how attractive will you feel as a bony, tired, skinny person, with sagging, droopy muscles?

#4. Setting short-term weight-loss goals instead of long ones.

If your thought process is, "I'll lose the weight quickly so I can go back to eating 'normally,'" guess what? You'll normally look like you started. The National Weight Control Registry suggests that dieters who successfully keep off lost weight for more than a year made their new eating style a habit by continuing the process they started even after they hit their correct weight. Funny how we do something successfully until we're successful, then revert. Dance with the one who brung ya.

#5. Assuming "healthy," "organic," "natural," "fat free," or "sugar free," equates to "low calorie."

Heed the almighty nutrition label! One half cup of "healthy, natural, organic" cereal might have 200 calories; think twice before consuming. Also, in order to keep the taste acceptable on many sugar-free foods, companies might add fat (or add sugar to fat-free foods.)

Bottom line? We engage in these behaviors because we're looking for the simplest road to our goal. That's normal; it's not like life is so easy that we need to complicate it. However, equally true – and certainly more frustrating – is that the less we adjust, the more unlikely we are to experience positive results. Change requires change.

My advice? Pick one thing; whether that be late night eating, start-and-stop dieting, or grazing from the office candy bowl. Be conscious, and alter it – even a little bit – whenever possible. Stick with that and repeat as necessary.

But most important, stop beating yourself up; after all, if guilt and shame were motivational, we'd all be skinny.

THE PERFECT
WEIGHT LOSS INVENTION!

I am going to make millions hawking a new weight loss contraption, which will revolutionize dieting! Every illustrious discovery is borne of the inferno of frustration; this is no exception.

As background, I used to pounce on my home scale several times a day; upon rising, each time I'm in the bathroom, before sleeping … blah, blah, blah. It's true; successful habit change requires regular self-monitoring, albeit "minute by minute" seemed a tad obsessive. So now I only allow myself per week one "unofficial" home weigh-in and one "official" check-in on the calibrated scale at my meeting. (Why at home? Um, I don't know. Just go with it, OK? It's how I am.)

First, make sure the two are in sync. In that process, I discovered my home scale records five pounds underweight, so if I tip 180 on it, my "real" weight is 185. In the event I cannot attend a meeting, I now can at least stay on track.

Two weeks ago, it flashes "177," meaning my "official" weight is 182, the long sought nirvana for which I've been aiming! I dance merrily about the bathroom in my skivvies (please don't focus on that image too long), exhilarated by the prospect of achieving "Goal" – a dream shortly dashed upon the rocks of despair when I later weigh in formally at 184. I, now a broken shell of a man, come despondently to the realization that my scale is at present off by seven pounds instead of what was five. OK, I can work with that.

Next week, determined to reach my happy place of 182, l again step tentatively upon the platform. The scale Gods smile upon me, answering my prayers with "175." Adding seven (no longer five) lets me arrive at the magic land of 182! Repeat skivvies dance. Repeat joyous exaltation. Repeat disappointment; as later, I again weigh – you got it –184.

There is no avoiding the conclusion my home scale is now ill. Somehow, its little computer brain has lost its bearings, and it is drifting further from true north with every passing day. Although I am losing a "virtual" two pounds per week, my actual weight remains static.

This is when opportunity, encased in such woeful tragedy; radiates unto me!

Why not manufacture a scale for uninspired dieters who merely want to feel good, but don't want to actually change? I could make a fortune! I could even eat a whole lot and tell everyone I'm losing weight, even when I can go longer snap shut my pants!

Therefore, I vow to create the "No Diet Scale." The first time someone stands on it, it records his actual weight, which it stores in memory. Then, each subsequent time he weighs himself, it automatically lowers that number by a small random amount. The more times you weigh, the more you lose!

What's best is the user gets to feel good, without all the pesky details of actually having to do anything! It's the perfect solution to the obesity problem. Since dieters will no longer feel trepidation about weighing themselves – quite the contrary, it will always be a reason to celebrate – more people will go on diets! Of course, they won't actually be losing anything – and I haven't figured out exactly how to handle it when the scale starts reading "negative weights," but my marketing team is working on those.

Pointing fingers at others

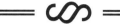

Cigarette smokers have long been relegated to the underclass of the social order. They are ostracized, even banished, from "polite society." This was hammered home to me recently while landing at Salt Lake City airport. Upon taxing to the terminal, the attendant takes to the microphone to make her customary proclamations: "Thank you for flying with us; we realize you have a choice of airlines. (I do?) Please don't remove your seat belt until the captain has pulled into the gate and, if you smoke, please do not do so until you arrive in the designated area inside the terminal."

Sure enough, literally smack-dab in the center of the terminal is an enclosed, glass-walled chamber where smokers light up and puff away to their heart's content. (That's probably a bad choice of expressions in light of the activity we're discussing.) What struck me was that through the grey misted air, they appeared as caged zoo animals, pacing in their restricted area, engaging in behaviors not accepted by the reminder of the population, while kept at a safe distance from those they could harm upon accidental release.

I found the whole thing to be incredibly sad.

Let me head off the armies of hacking militant, wheezing smokers who, even before they have finished reading this piece, are racing to computers to fire off angry missives about how I am insulting them. My comments are not as much levied at those who have chosen to engage in this habit as much as at the society that determines what is appropriate and what is not. Mores change and smoking, once considered "the cat's meow," is now considered gauche, existing in a strange societal limbo – scorned yet legal.

I am allergic to tobacco smoke. Moreover, having previously lived with a smoker, the stench that permeated and saturated everything from clothing to carpeting invoked regularly my gag reflex. So, I'm A-OK with the act being isolated. Yet, what is not tolerable to me is that it appears that we – the "Proper Members of Society" – are forever judging others in a misguided effort to feel better about ourselves, while ignoring our own annoying foibles.

Civility's spotlight, although not shifting from the nicotine user, has lately expanded to include the overweight. As with users of cigarettes, behind their backs, we shake our heads and whisper to our "normal" friends, "It's a shame that they don't take care of themselves. I'd never let myself look like that." We wag our fingers and click our tongues, satisfied that we are "better than that."

It's probably human nature to try and elevate oneself by putting down others. I know in my lesser moments that I am not immune. However, it seems that each and everyone of us has habits of which we would not want exposed to bright sunlight. Creating new sub-classes determined by what one eats or smokes is divisive, and we've got plenty of that going around.

I've got bad habits. You do too. It's not a reflection of self-worth; it is a method by which each of us is trying to make it through the day without collapsing under the weight of its stress. I'm not advocating abandoning personal responsibility and "let it all hang out;" quite the contrary. The process of growth is the cycle of "identify, adjust, and modify." It seems if each of us spent a tad more energy striving to be an example instead of a judge, it could alter the atmosphere just enough that we wouldn't need a cigarette – or bag of chips – quite as often.

IT'S NOT THE NUMBER,
IT'S THE BENEFITS

Obesity is by no means only a difficulty in the U.S. of A. As more of our planet has found its way to a more affluent lifestyle, faster food, and less exercise, the collective global waistline has expanded. As of this time, approximately 1.6 billion people on planet Earth are overweight. Of those, 400 million (more than the entire population of our country) are obese. Despite the urgency, the problem grows. In five years, it is estimated that more than 2.3 billion people will be overweight, with almost 3/4 of a billion being obese. (Note: the standard definition of "obese" is more than 20% above normal body weight or having a body mass index – "BMI" – over 30. A normal healthy BMI is considered to be between 21 and 25.)

Let's put this in perspective. When the baby boomers started being born shortly after World War II, the entire population inhabiting this third rock from the sun was 2.3 billion. Therefore, if we lived in 1947, and we were facing this same predicament, every single, solitary, person would need to be on a diet.

While we're playing "interesting facts to quote at cocktail parties," let me toss you another: NOBODY diets to lose weight.

Huh?

Anybody who has ever tried to trim a pound from a pudgy mid-section, whether by changing the way she eats or by increasing her exercise level (or both), has not embarked upon that path to weigh a certain number or to drop X pounds. She launched into the process to achieve the BENEFITS that the weight loss will provide. Lifestyle change – in this case eating healthier – is simply the vehicle she has chosen to obtain an improved life; henceforth referred to as the "benefit."

Moreover, how she chooses to define "better" is up to her: healthier, happier, more attractive, self-confident, more active, or anything else that tickles her fancy. But the bottom line remains that weight loss unto itself is not what drove the change, the results of it set the motion forward.

It might seem like we're picking nits, but the cool thing about understanding benefits is that we can see them almost immediately, and that's inspiring. However, waiting for the scale's number to drop can appear to take forever, making the process feel much worse and more difficult than necessary. Restated, if I focus on benefits, the effort it's taking to lose weight seems lessened.

For example, even if I am just starting my diet today, several benefits kick in even before one ounce has been lost. There is a sense of relief about overcoming procrastination, pride for moving forward on a goal, and my energy will probably spike due to the healthier combination of foods I'm now consuming. Conversely, if my sole measurement of success is a number on a scale, there's one long road to hoe before I get any strokes from the process.

If I focus on the benefits received, which are plenty; rather than the effort it requires, which in reality is not really that much; not only will the end results be the same, but life will most likely be more rewarding and fun. Dare I say it: yet another benefit of being healthy.

Unfortunate episode at the clothing store

===== ∽ =====

It is the night before I fly to a speaking engagement and I am in the all-too-familiar pattern of attempting to stuff too much clothing into a too-small carry-on bag. Since I do this with regularity, I have learned to plot out my week's apparel on a grid, so I can bring as few items as possible while assuring those who see me speak on Wednesday, won't be shocked by me wearing the same clothing Thursday. (Does one spell "anal-retentive" with or without the hyphen?) This procedure also helps determine the minimum amount of clothing to lug. In this process, I realized that a plain black pair of dress pants could serve double duty. Alas, not being the owner of such – I make an emergency run to the clothing store.

A dapper gentleman greets me, "How can I help you sir?"

"Black dress pants please."

"Which size?"

"Thirty-four by 30," I reply. I know this well. Personally, I call it them "32 WLD," which means "32 while lying down," but since he's a professional in the clothing business, he probably refers to them as "34." I shall – in deference to being in his store – speak his language.

He scopes me out and says, "No, you're a 36."

Sucking in my stomach – and now extremely self conscious – I counter, defensively, "No, I'm a 34, been a 34 for 15 years."

Yet, inside, my ego is rapidly turning to jelly, "Am I putting on weight? Maybe I'm bloated? Does this make me look fat?" Oy, the horrible maelstrom of verbal cacophony blowing about in my gray matter! I want to shriek, "Don't you dare tell me what size I am! I am a professional dieter. I can list the calories, fat, fiber, and sugar content of every food ever invented. Go ahead, test me!" Feeling mall security would not take kindly to a raving maniac in bulging britches, I opt to keep closed my pie hole.

Oblivious to the paranoia he has foisted upon my shallow, weak – apparently chubby – ego, he lifts his arms so I can take in the full view of his thinner-than-me waistline and points to himself, "I wear a 34." As an afterthought, realizing one doesn't want to tell a customer he's looking tubby, he quickly appends, "These pants are cut really small." Too late buddy, the damage has been done.

He hands me a 36 and I plod, a broken, rotund man, to the fitting room where I pull them over my legs. Hallelujah! Great day in Heaven, I'm practically swimming in them! A choir of well-tailored angels sings from above, I am validated! Yet, I must also be vindicated.

Tugging my pants upward with one hand, like a gen-exer hefting up too-baggy trousers, I strut boldly into the middle of the store, pointing at my waist with my free hand and triumphantly proclaiming for all to hear, "Ah-hem! These are waaaay too large."

He eyes my droopy drawers, respond with, "I think they fit well. However, if you want something smaller, we can do that."

Suggestion to clothing store employees: Never tell your customer they are larger than they say they say they are. If I want to squeeze my 62-inch waist into a 29-inch pair of jeans, let me try. Simply clear the patrons out of the store in anticipation of when the button explodes.

FEAR OF SUCCESS

There are few reasons why we do not achieve our dreams.

Yes, there are "acts of God." Philosophically, one might even accept fate or destiny as insurmountable barriers. Yet, aside from those, the immense majority of people living lives of quiet desperation reside there because of what's going on in their minds more than on our planet. With credit to Walt Kelly, "We have met the enemy and he is us." We – not others – are more times than not, our worst adversaries.

I mean this not in a condescending, judgmental manner, as one might hear from no-nonsense hyper-achievers, "Just pull yourself up from the bootstraps, suck it in, and get it done. Don't be such a wimp!" One cannot change years of brain wave patterns in the same manner in which he switches on or off a light. Negative thoughts today – click – positive henceforth. My objective today is also not designed to illustrate how messed up we are; I don't think that's true, we're all doing the best we know how to do.

With appropriate disclaimers admitted, if we accept that we are standing in our own way, it begs the question, "Why would we do that?" Why do we NOT reach further, dream larger, and believe better?

The primary answer is: Fear; Fear of Success, and its dastardly sibling, Fear of Failure.

These concepts are tossed about often than a well-worn basketball in a high school gym, yet rarely do we take the time to understand the difference between the two. For in doing so, we might be able to get past them.

Usually, Fear of Success is an apprehension that achieving one's goals could generate future events unforeseen or out of one's control and we won't know what to do with them. For example, if I lose weight, members of the opposite sex might look at me differently. I might need to deal with flirting, or even sexual tensions, that – until now – have been kept at bay by the extra layers in which I can (literally and figuratively) hide. Another illustration could be that I worry friends who currently socialize with me around food (such as going out to lunch) might no longer feel comfortable doing so. What will we do then? Will I lose friendships? Will I become lonely?

Fear of Success's baseline concern is I might not like the way things are right now, but at least I know how to handle them. Change them and it could be worse.

Fear of Failure, far more common, is being scared that my goals are really just empty pipe dreams. The regret in attempting it – and failing – would be so much more devastating than the conditions in which I now find myself, that I'd rather just stay put. In other words, "If I don't do anything, I can't fail and therefore, I won't be disappointed. As it stands currently, at least I have my fantasy to comfort me. I am unwilling to risk those."

Fear is a normal, sometimes even healthy, emotion. Like a fortress it can keep out what might harm us – or, as a cage, it can prevent us from getting what we want.

ONE PERFECT DAY

I fly a great deal. Well, that's not exactly accurate; I am in airplanes a great deal. They fly. I merely constrict my five-feet-eight-inches of body into about three-feet-seven-inches of space for four hours 18 minutes of discomfort, late arrivals, and poor service. It's a privilege for which I pay a great deal of money.

To alleviate the numbness in my limbs, I think of walking. However scrambling and stumbling over three other contorted travelers to stagger sloth like down a scrawny center aisle following a unhurriedly moving food cart with attendants lobbing overpriced "box meals" to ravenous twisted travelers doesn't sound advantageous. Therefore, I read.

One of the airlines on which I frequently endure travel has a regular feature in their magazine. It lays out how to spend a few "perfect days" in an exotic city. For example, "three perfect days in Paris," or "four perfect days in Bangkok." They have yet to list "six perfect days in Eureka" but I am sure it is soon to be.

My internal recovering perfectionist is intrigued by the very concept of a "perfect day." What would it be like? For that matter, is it even possible? And, of course, since all things in my life filter through the screen of dieting, my thoughts turned toward, "What would it be like to be perfect on my diet for one week?"

Of course, counter-intuitively, it's thoughts like those that actually trigger failure. By expecting to be "perfect," an impossibility, one sets himself up to "blow it," a human experience. The perfectionist, after slipping on the path to attain the stated goal of 100 percent, says, "Well, as long as I blew it, I might as well really blow it. I'll start again tomorrow;" actually remaining stagnant in the pursuit of his goal. I believe "perfectionism" is an excuse to avoid doing the actual, ongoing, daily effort required to simply get "better."

Therefore, with those as my beliefs, I quickly dismissed the concept of "seven perfect days" doing anything. But, I thought, "What about "three perfect days?" Three seems doable; at least it did, until I realized I have to eat out a few times this week. Should I put butter on my roll at my favorite Italian restaurant; have I then abandoned the sought-after grail of perfection? For that matter, is even going to an Italian restaurant considered "failing?" What happens if I have an extra glass of wine? Now what? Where does one draw the line?

No, too much effort to be perfect to do three days. What about one?

Could I do absolutely everything I need to do for one complete turn of the Earth without making even the teensy-weensiest error? Could I write down everything I eat? Could I prepare all my foods in the healthiest fashion possible? Would I weigh and measure every morsel that entered my mouth? Would I take time to sit and reflect on whether I'm actually being driven by hunger or appetite before chowing down? Would I? Could I? Will I? Only for one day.

Nah. I know me; it ain't gonna happen.

But, know what? Just the thought of how "good" I could be caused me to think about what I was doing that day. I didn't have a perfect day; but I had a darn-well great one. Should I have more days like that than not, it would feel like a luxury vacation my entire life.

THE TOOL BOX

Building a life is constructing a house. Create a solid foundation. Once achieved, place down brick one. Secure it. Add additional ones nearby or on top. Check stability. Repeat until desired results are obtain. Of course, many times the "curb appeal" of our domicile is not exactly what we thought we were building, appearing as happenstance. Walls are crooked. The garden has weeds. The entire thing seems in a state of.

"Why is my marriage a mess?" "How come I weigh so much?" "Will I ever save enough to retire?" These are all questions a life-contractor might ask when examining a "dwelling" that appears not at all as the architect envisioned.

Nonetheless, each structure is built to our exacting specifications. Granted, sometimes "stuff" outside of our control happens. Earthquakes, illness, even political forces, can interfere with well-developed plans. Yet, the underlying truth for the vast majority of us is that the vast majority of time, we are where we are because of what we have done so far. Want to live differently? Act differently. New materials and a modernization might be the order of the day.

It seems like a simple solution. Yet the unhappy truth is that to accomplish that also takes planning. It is essential that we examine each and every brick; come to a decision as to whether or not it's functional, as well as which others rely upon it for their support. Then, and only then, can we choose whether we simply demolish it or must substitute it with another. Of course, we can even retain some exactly where they rest.

Unfortunately, too often, we take the tact of a demolitionist and attempt to simply "start over." That's folly, oft-time guaranteed to fail, as we cannot just knock everything over and start anew. Those bricks labeled "how I treat my family" or "what I do for a living" are cemented to those emblazoned, "sit rather than walk," "eat to handle stress," and "chips instead of vegetables." Starting from scratch is the metaphorical option of being homeless. I might not like where I live, but it beats the street. "There's always tomorrow."

Let's presume however, that we take a more long-term line of attack and begin the careful disassembly and future reassembly. There is yet that other level: that pesky slab upon which everything rests. If we erect the most magnificent mansion rooted in a plot of sand, further problems are ensured. In this cautionary fable, that foundation consists of thoughts and feelings. Our actions, the bricks, are built upon inextricably intertwined thoughts and feelings. Should they not be able to direct well our actions, we shall yet again be housed in a hovel.

This begs an urgent question: Do we control our thoughts and feelings or do they control us? In effect, are we victims to the synaptic firings and hormone-driven changes of affect; or do we create them to serve our needs? Who is the master – and who is servant?

If we believe that we have little or no control over what enters our consciousness – in effect, they just "happen" – we are forever at the whim of those electrical impulses and influences. Any plan at any time can be immediately disrupted by seemingly random fluctuations pulsing though our system.

Conversely, if we can accept that our thoughts and our feelings can be developed, guided, molded, and in some cases, even controlled; we are given the most powerful tools imaginable. With those in the toolbox, there is no limit as to what we can construct.

THE FINAL THING

I am ablaze! I figured out the final thing I have to do to get my act together! It's a new dawn; heaven has opened wide; the path is clear; I am complete! Just picturing it makes me so excited I can barely sit still!

But, here's the thing about the thing. You can't just jump into it, you know? I mean, after all, something as grandiose as this requires forethought and meticulous planning. That's why I'll be successful where others wouldn't! See, I have a handle on the fact you just don't launch willy-nilly hither and yon down the boulevard into something as pressing, essential, and life-altering as a thing like this can be. You better be primed, that's what I have to say.

And I am! Nothing will hold me back! I'm getting my ducks in a row; putting my house in order; stepping one foot in front of the other; yes sirree Bob! I'm figuring out the flawless, exact method to ensure I do it just so. Don't want to take my shot and blow it. You hear me, don't ya' bro?

In days gone by, I tended to rush without forethought into critical decisions. Now, being wiser, I know first elicit support. It's slowing me down somewhat because – well, I don't mean to brag – but I'm a pretty popular guy, you know? I have friends on top of friends; want to make sure they're all on board. I've called several, emailed buckets more; even posted it on Facebook. That's the way to build consensus though. It's time-consuming, but when you're a forward-thinking guy like me, you appreciate that's the price of success. Slow and steady; tortoise and hare; you know how it goes.

But after that, watch out, boy howdy! After you heed your peeps, you chart your actions. Those of us in the know value that if you write down the objectives, line 'em out, set 'em in motion; they're far more likely to happen. Measure twice, cut once; right? So, I'll take a few days for a secluded personal retreat where I compile the input, and write, write, write!

I bet you're asking, "But won't your wife be there?"

See! I don't mean to be cold but this is why this thing will work for me and it might not for you. You're not thinking like a winner my friend. Remember, I did that consensus thing already; my mate's on board. She realizes how key this is; we're a well-oiled team. She'll give me the room to engage in the vital, necessary planning something like this entails. Yep, team-building equals success; that's my creed.

Of course, I've got to figure out how much to spend on a getaway this vital; so, back to that good old support network for more input, and additional advice. Then, breakdown the replies, verify the up-shot; and run it back up the flagpole to corroborate it's correct. If I made a mistake – hard to believe, huh? – I do it again.

I know what you're thinking, "There's a lot of activity but no action." See! Readin' you like a book, aren't I? I saw that coming.

What you're missing is this is so fool-proof that someday, when all the lights are on green, the results have been filtered, costs analyzed, benefits weighed, potential evaluated, course plodded, outcomes made clear – and everyone supports me, I'll be do the thing perfectly! At that point, it's lead, follow, or out of my way!

OBESE CHILDREN
AND BULLYING

It was lousy growing up fat. Nothing was more degrading than buying my clothes in the "husky" section. Okay, maybe showering in front of a bunch of guys after high school P.E. was worse... or, wait, never dating ... or, wait a second, here's one: being teased behind my back – and for that matter – to my face... or, well ... I guess there are countless things that suck about being a fat kid.

A recent study shows that obese children in grades three through six are more likely to be bullied than children of a normal weight. Teen suicide due to bullying – an absolutely horrifying thought – has tragically been in the news a great deal, raising awareness of the psychological impact of constant harassment. Now we discover that that it begins at an early age, with overweight children as the primary target.

Based on my own memories, I didn't find this to be news. However, I had assumed, or maybe naively hoped, that things had changed. Not so, as researchers at the University of Michigan surveyed over 800 children ages eight to 11. In the third grade, 15 percent of the children were overweight and 17 percent were obese. A quarter of the students admitted to being bullied; with 45 percent of the mothers reporting that her child had been bullied for his or her weight. The odds of being bullied were 63 percent higher for children who were obese than their classmates of a normal weight, and bullies did not discriminate based on gender or economic status. Overweight boys were just as likely as girls to be bullied, and even those with good social skills weren't spared.

"I thought maybe (good social skills) would protect obese kids from being bullied. But no matter how we ran and re-ran the analysis, the link between being obese and being bullied remained," said Dr. Julie Lumeng, lead researcher. She is concerned that the perception surrounding obesity is that it's caused by a lack of exercise and overeating when the underlying condition is often driven by other factors. "Many times, children who are not good at dealing with their emotions become emotional eaters," she explained, noting, "we really need to work on changing this view of what causes obesity."

My first response to this story was sadness, bringing me back to my own early days. The study suggested that we not only need to encourage healthy eating habits for young children, but also need to set a good example by refraining from making negative comments about people who are overweight. Children of course, are mirrors of us and they pick up our attitude, which results in bullying behavior. In effect, we indirectly teach our children to bully.

However, there is a bigger picture. We need to remember that each and every person has habits about which he or she is not proud. The difference is that if overeating is the habit, it cannot be hidden. It is on display for all to view.

Smoke too much but hide well? No one knows. Have trouble with anger management but it doesn't leak into public? We won't judge you. Yet, eat too many fries and not exercise enough, and everyone's got a comment. Seems to me that if we each paid a little more attention to our own issues, we'd all be happier and healthier.

Maybe, when I've achieved complete perfection, I can judge others. However, I don't see that happening soon.

Lose ten pounds – and your health – in three days

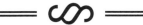

Searching the worldwide wacky web I stumble across: *"Lose ten pounds in three days!"* Intrigued, I find myself on a discussion page for a "fantastic new diet." Let's review, shall we? (Warning: If you are capable of rational thought, tread carefully.)

DAY ONE

Breakfast:
Black coffee or tea
half cup grapefruit
one slice toast
two tablespoons peanut butter

Lunch:
half cup tuna
one slice toast
coffee

Dinner:
seven slices meat
one cup string beans
beets
one small apple
one cup vanilla ice cream.

DAY TWO

Breakfast:
One egg
half banana
one slice toast
coffee

Lunch:
one cup cottage cheese
three saltine crackers

Dinner:
two hot dogs
one cup of broccoli
half cup carrots
cup of vanilla ice cream

Day three is a virtual repeat. Beyond that, instructions include, *"Do not vary or substitute foods. In three days you will lose ten pounds and then you can eat normal food, but do not overdo it. After four days of normal eating, start back on the diet."*

Let's wade right in, shall we? Aside from the obvious best advice about dieting anywhere, "Don't overdo it;" who dreamt this up? I mean any diet that requires hot dogs has to be a joke. They – and the ice cream – were probably tossed in simply to prevent one from going bonkers while protectively hunkering over and guarding the three saltine crackers and one miserly beet.

And, as near as I can tell, one consumes only about 800 calories per day. Should anyone starve themselves with such a low caloric intake, while eating virtually anything, such as marshmallows, sugar, and ice cream, yes, they'd lose weight. Of course, they'd lose teeth, muscle mass, and any chance at good health. That does seems secondary to some, as one person posted, "I lost eight pounds. I don't believe in the whole 'science' thing yadda yadda, but it was a plan that got me to eat fewer calories."

Okay, Scott, take a deep breath, don't let your head explode; you might need it. Maybe it was her lack of calories, but, "I don't believe the whole science thing?" Where does one even go from there? I don't believe the whole "gravity" thing or I'm not subscribing to the whole "earth is round" thing? I guess health is so yesterday when you can fit in a size two, right? I mean, let's get our priorities straight, shall we?

In fairness, many comments did label it unhealthy. However, one endorsed it enthusiastically, "THIS DIET DOES WORK! As a wrestler, my weight is very important. Last year, I put on ten pounds. I was scared of not making weight so I gave this a try. On the third day, I was nine pounds lighter."

He concludes – get ready for it, "I am now around 25 pounds overweight, so I am going to do it again."

See, there it is! If it worked so well, you would not be "doing it again," you'd still be "doing it" from before. At the risk of being the proverbial broken record, (repeat after me): "Its NOT about weight, it's about healthy habits!" One can be at his right weight and be unhealthy. Yet, if you're healthy, you'll naturally be at your correct weight. No matter what you eat, the weight will exist until one one adopts a balanced lifestyle: Eat a little less, add healthier foods, walk a little more, and avoid seeking a quick fix.

WHERE DOES SUCCESS BEGIN?

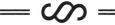

When do I get to call myself "successful," and like the movie character, Rocky, stand proudly on high, arms outstretched over my head, surveying my accomplishments below?

Does that brand apply only after my entire, complete, absolute goal has been achieved? Upon reaching that summit and overcoming each and every barrier, do I then – and only then – transition from "failure" to "success?" I mean, somewhere, at some indefinable point along the journey – even if I were not able to travel the road as far or quickly as originally planned – it would still seem that I am entitled to call whatever I accomplished, "victory."

It goes without saying that upon 100 percent accomplishment of my goal I am "successful." But in reality, success starts prior to completion. On the thousand-mile journey, should I fall short by one step, we would call it a triumph. So, if 99.9 percent is "victory;" can we not stretch it to 99.8 percent – or even 98.4 percent? Where do we draw the line before rewards are appropriate?

This is not merely an ethereal discussion without real-life implication, similar to "how many angels can dance on the head of a pin." These terms we toss about: "success," "failure," "victory," "defeat;" are bound, Gordian-knot style into our psyche. They manipulate us emotionally; and it is what we feel – far beyond what we think – that drives action. The totality of those actions we call "life." Therefore, these powerful words, and their associated feelings, determine the quality of our life, and whether we are "successful" or a "failure." The cycle begins and ends with words. Therefore what we choose to say matters to the highest degree.

Refraining from the celebration and recognition of the small successes peppered throughout our daily lives will not drive us harder to accomplish our goals. Counter intuitively, the opposite is true, to be truly successful, it is essential that we find small victories often and regularly. Success – with a capital "S" – is not borne unto its own. Rather, it is formed via a series of small "s" successes, each allowing the opportunity for reflection, evaluation, and celebration.

As an example, many (including myself) herald my seventy-pound weight loss as success. Yet I actually only lost one pound – and repeated the process 70 times, constantly reminding myself how great it was for every accomplishment that stuck, instead of – as I had done in former days – holding back congratulations until the end of the line, which I never reached.

To believe that, "Nothing short of my goal is success" is a noble, but misguided, thought, as it keeps us focused always on the distance yet to travel, rather than the day-to-day accomplishments already achieved. That, simply stated, is discouraging. Discouragement is the cement that holds us stagnant.

Once I could accept that each pound, or every meal, or even getting back on track after falling off, was success, I began enjoying the fruits of my efforts and looked forward with anticipation, rather than dread. This drove me to push forward, eventually reaching my goal.

Success is interwoven in every accomplishment, no matter how small; it's much more prevalent than we notice. Furthermore, we will only achieve the big goals when we acknowledge our victory over the little ones.

It's hard to be positive

I can uncover the dark cloud behind any silver lining. No matter how undersized the trigger, with just a little time – and a whole lot of paranoia – I can blow it up into a full-scale panic attack. I am no amateur; I have developed this ability beyond the level of a fine art; and I am able to apply it to any aspect of life with equal proficiency.

For example, sometimes I walk from one room to another and forget why I was going to the new location. It happens, you know? I'm busy; I had a spark of an idea which didn't lock it into the right location in my jam-packed brain and suddenly, there I am standing in the center of my living room staring at the wall painting, befuddled, questioning myself, "Now, why did I want to come in here?"

I could simply laugh it off, attributing it to the "human condition." But, no, not me! I use this minor brain-blurp as a springboard to convince myself that I have the first symptom of long-term memory loss, providing me an opportunity to freak out about my vanishing faculties, forgotten youth, and the inevitable bleak fate which awaits us all, apparently much closer than I anticipated. From there, I spin into a tornado of dread and fright, racing to the internet, researching Alzheimer's, dementia, and senility. It goes without saying that once one enters the festering, moldy hallways of the worldwide web, countless unimaginable horrific ailments are all now on parade, many of which can now be attributed to this very circumstance. I might as well give up, accept the inescapable, collapse to the carpet, hold my knees tight to my chest, while rocking back and forth, and babbling incoherently.

All right, I'm really not that bad; I'm taking poetic license. Please don't send me referrals for therapists. This is what we call the "set up" making a broader point.

Research has actually proven that humans are "hard-wired" to assume things will go cattywumpus rather than not. Given the opportunity to attribute a random event to either good new or bad, we will usually assume the road has more potholes than flat patches.

In ancient times, it made sense to assume the worst. Primitive hunter-gatherers would go into an idyllic serene valley. The optimists would find this yet one more reason to relax, breathe deeply, catch fish, lie in the sun, and assume the best. Their counterparts, pessimists, spent every waking moment distressing about any type of calamity, turning their existence into an unending backbreaking chain of toil and labor, always one step shy of collapse.

Said the optimists to the pessimists, "Relax, take a load off. Don't worry so much."

Said the pessimists in reply, "Are you kidding? This whole thing could come apart at any second. You'll be sorry." With that, they'd turn on their heals and race into the hills, in search of protection from the impending, unforeseen catastrophe.

As it happens, while the pessimists are away engaged in their grueling method of survival, the river overtops its banks, drowns the unaware optimists, and leaves only the pessimists – who therefore became our ancestors. The trait of hard-luck survival has been passed down ever since.

Anticipation and planning surely have their place. Yet, it's equally important to realize that worry is interest on a debt not yet owed. After all, if worry made things better, I single-handedly would be able to correct everything.

It's going be what it's going be, enjoy it while it's here.

Ending the dysfunctional relationship

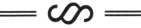

We've all had them, those relationships that didn't quite work out as expected.

I just ended one and I share my saga as a cautionary tale, because although you're similar to me, you're probably not inclined to air your dirty laundry in the newspaper. Therefore, I shall throw myself on the sword for all of us – for every person facing weight issues who has developed an unnatural attraction to his bathroom scale. Oh sure, we've tried to kick the habit, but every time, we gained weight.

Speaking for myself, I think I got too involved too quickly. I couldn't handle being alone. I'd check my weight first thing in the morning and as the last activity before retiring at night. I'd monitor myself before and after every meal and each time I visited the restroom.

I began to feel like there should be a support group for those of us excessively and overly fixated with the number attached to our weight.

"Hi, my name is Scott. I'm a bathroom scale addict."

(Group response): "Hello Scott."

Not meaning to make too much light of a serious situation, but there were times when it seemed like I couldn't go for hours, let alone days, without rushing to see my lovely placed patiently on the bathroom floor, gently flicking the on switch with my foot, hopping lightly on to the flat white platform, and awaiting the calming rush (or abject depression) of what the flashing red LED screen would proclaim.

To be even closer, I envisioned a device whereby one could insert special plates into the soles of his shoes, so with each footfall his weight would be calculated. Then, similar to those electronic stock tickers that crawl across the bottom of the TV screen, a series of numbers telling you your up-to-the-moment, right-at-that-second weight would parade across your field of view in specially made goggles connected via Bluetooth to your shoes. Therefore, with each step, you have an instant standing on whether your weight was up, down, or holding. Like some sort of crazed day-trader, you could make split-second decisions on how to adjust what you're doing to maximize your dieting return.

Can we say, "Unhealthy obsession?" (OK, I wasn't that severe; but I was trending.)

I was discussing how despondent my relationship was making me, after an unfortunate event when it had foretold of a heavy and tragic weight gain. Yet upon standing on the "official" scale at my weekly meeting, I was bowled over to find out I had in reality lost two pounds! My scale, my beloved, had betrayed me. I felt so used, so abandoned, so confused.

My buddy chimed in, "Why don't you just stay away from that scale? It seems to be a harmful relationship."

Just stay off the scale, leave it alone, shut the emotional door behind, and walk into the distance? What a concept. Skip all the fussing and frustrations associated with the ups and downs of my daily weight and lead a normal healthy life? Could that be possible? Can I do it?

So, I mustered up my courage, took a deep breath, and bid adieu to our past. I know it wasn't about her, it was more about me, but our goals were no longer compatible. It was time to end it.

I still think back fondly to those twenty-seven-times-a-day rendez-vous on the tile floor, but I know I'm better off alone. I don't need a relationship that's quite so heavy any longer.

Accepting what comes

When my mother celebrated her 70th birthday (I was a mere lad of 40), I asked her if she felt any different from when she was in her thirties. She pondered the question for a moment and replied, "No not really. I look in the mirror and it's obvious I'm not who I was – and the parts don't always work they way they used to; causing me to slow down. I've got some annoying aches and pains. But, big picture? Inside, I feel like I always have."

I've since queried other seniors about whether they feel "elderly." Whether the respondent was 70, 80 – I even got to ask someone who was 99 – the answer was almost always identical, "I pretty much feel like I always have.'"

This begs a question: At what point do we accept that we're "old" – or at least "older?"

This somewhat gloomy line of thought has been prompted by the realization that if we come with a warranty, I fear mine lapsed recently. Since I hit "double nickels," seemingly all at once, my parts are sore, not working well, acting quirky, or just plain out of sorts. I have pains in places where I did not even know I had places. I am continuously complaining about some dang cramp or soreness, which I do not like doing, and I assure you that is definitely NOT me. My foremost fear is that I shall soon devolve into a cranky, wrinkly, grey-haired, curmudgeonly man-creature, who brandishes his cane at the clouds and rants at the heavens about the unfairness of life.

This is even more troublesome because I'm doing my bit to forestall that unhappy outcome. I walk regularly, eat well, take vitamins, don't stress (except about this), attend Yoga classes, ride a bike; and – I might point out – I'm a heck of a nice guy! One would therefore assume with such a powerful curriculum vitae of healthy habits and proper outlook, I should easily surpass 125 years before I even go so far as to pull a muscle.

My loving wife has (gently) pointed out that I'm "not as young as I was," and these symptoms could be interrelated. However I refuse to accept it's the aging process. I'll age gracefully (whatever the heck that means) but will not go gently, so off to the doctor I go where I inventory everything that's sore, bruised, inconsistent, nasty, gnarly, gross, inflated, swollen, hot, cold, flat, red, or black and blue. He types and listens; studies the computer; clarifies a few details; and then says, "I've got good news and bad news."

"What's the good news?"

"There's nothing serious; no need to worry."

Sigh of relief… "What's the bad news?"

"Your wife is right."

"But Doc," I proclaim, "I take good care of myself," as if that argument will cause him to reverse the prognosis.

"Yes, you do. But at your age, things don't recover as quickly. It would be worse if you weren't doing what you're doing."

So, that's it? Sounds like an attitude adjustment might be in order.

They say this is a "normal process" and I'm obviously I'm in it. In all honesty, I do enjoy the peace, self-confidence, and serenity at this stage of life. My marriage is wonderful. My friendships are close. And, overall, I am happy with where I am. That's what really matters.

Placed in that perspective, I can handle a few bumps, bruises and a periodic cramp, as long as it's "nothing serious." I really do think I'm fine with that.

RUMORS ABOUT
THE AGING BRAIN

John Mellencamp, whom I consider to be Norman Rockwell with a rock and roll beat, is one of my favorite musicians. On his album "Lonesome Jubilee" is the song "The Real Life," dealing with life's changes and adjusting to what comes. The last verse contains these lyrics:

"But something happens/When you reach a certain age/Particularly to those ones that are young at heart/It's a lonely proposition when you realize/That's there's less days in front of the horse/Than riding in the back of this cart" (I so appreciate the song that I won't even point out the glaring screw-up in grammar. Am I magnanimous or what?)

With that as set up, I lately am more and more focused on what it's like to continue down the path on which we each find ourselves. I don't mean in some "Oh-my-God-we're-all-going-to-die!" end-of-the-world manner. Rather, I would compare it more to studying an owner's manual. I've got this body, this machine; I want to know how it works so I can experience it to its fullest. And I better learn about it before it's too late.

One of the less pleasant perceptions many of us share is that we become more forgetful once we hit middle age; we don't remember our glasses are on top of our heads; or we climb stairs and forget why we wanted to go upstairs in the first place. It's puzzling, frustrating, and, at times, a bit frightening. To the rescue comes a new book, "The Secret Life of the Grown-Up Brain" by Barbara Strauch, whereby she points out that there's little reason to accept the conventional wisdom that we suffer a decline in brainpower as we age.

"We're wasting the best brains of our lives. We should appreciate them," says she. ("Here! Here!" says I.) Contrary to popular belief, our brain powers up and grows in cognitive ability as we age, reorganizing itself and using more of its parts to solve problems. Studies are proving that peak brain performance is actually between 40 and 68 years of age, what most people call "middle age." However, even in our early 70s, the average age when cognitive decline is seen, many of us just keep cruising along without such symptoms. Even while the brain slows down, the growth in cognitive depth and reasoning power causes a "net gain" during this period of our lives, Strauch said.

We're brought up to think it's going to be doom and gloom once we hit empty nest. Yet, says Strauch, the proverbial "mid-life crisis" only affects about five percent of us. Beyond that, we denizens of the land of middle age actually feel we have a greater sense of control over our lives. That's a blessing all by itself, but scientists have linked that emotional well-being with mental alertness and a lower risk of Alzheimer's disease. And it doesn't stop there. The aging brain appears to selectively focus on positive memories rather than on stress or negativity, according to Stanford psychologist Laura Carstensen. As it turns out, research has found out that the due to the brain's ability to better regular emotion, we experience increased feelings of well-being between the ages of 40 and 60.

Of course, there are things we can do to help keep our brains healthy longer including exercising, trying new mental activities, eating in a healthy fashion, and minding our moods. It seems keeping a positive attitude is surprisingly important to our gray matter. After reading about what happens during these years, that's not as difficult to do as it was previously.

Advice to husbands and other significant others

People contact me about my column. Many want to share their thoughts or feelings about what I have written. Most times it's by email, once in awhile by telephone, and periodically in person.

Some folks seem drawn to anyone in the media as moths go to light. This is flattering but can be, at times, well, just plain weird. I've been approached about government meat conspiracies, high fructose corn syrup alternative energy systems, even a faster-than-light engine (no, I don't know how it was tied to my column). If cornered publicly with such theories, I momentarily feign attention, smile awkwardly, mumble an apologetic excuse about "a guy I'm supposed to meet," and carefully; very, very slowly; back away.

There are those who offer to me the secret "they" don't want "us" to know about weight loss – for a price of course. I am cynical about "secrets they don't want us know." For one, who are "they?" Secondly, why would they deem you to be the ultimate messenger of such vital intelligence? Moreover, are you putting us in harm's way by passing it along? I would feel miserable knowing that – although I now lose weight quicker – it was at the cost of your life. Actually, I'd feel so darn guilty; I'd probably eat too much, gain back my weight and make your magnanimous (albeit mercenary) gesture to have been in vain.

What affects me most are those seeking counsel. I'm not a therapist; heck, I'm not even sure I could be "Dear Abby." But if my words touch someone so deeply that they seek me out for guidance, I'll do my best.

Some conventional wisdom portrays my gender as uncaring, stoic, non-feeling, self-absorbed louts more concerned with cold beer and hot chicks than a supportive relationship, a strong family, and an engaged life. If you're still holding that stereotype – some unsolicited advice: let it go. If your man is truly like that, maybe you ought to let him go. Just sayin'…

A caring husband, asking for advice on how he can help his wife, is a common focus of emails I receive. They usually go something like: "I love my wife no matter how much she weighs. I think she's beautiful. But I want her to be happy and healthy. I'm concerned because I think her weight has gotten to a point that it's harming her health. What can I do to make sure she stays on her diet?"

If you're in that place, here's my best, most sincere advice. Understand that NO ONE can make ANYONE do ANYTHING, at least not in a loving supportive relationship. All any of us can do is put out there how we feel, express what we desire, and then hope they will respond.

People who need to lose weight know it. Many times, they feel embarrassed because they've promised to do so so many times that the perceived risk of humiliation yet again is more painful than what they weigh. Often, they simply don't believe they can do it "one more time." Sometimes, they're even afraid that if they do, they'll lose their relationships.

Your (albeit well-intentioned) push will move her in one direction: away from you.

So, what to do? Be honest. Tell her how you feel. Tell her you're concerned. Remind her you love her and you'd like her to be healthy; and if she wants help, you're there.

Then love her for who she is, let go as much as you can, and be there if and when she asks for help.

Some of what we do is obvious

Sitting at my usual table, at my usual coffee house, at the usual time, I'm not sure I "read" my newspaper, per se. I glance at an article, absorb a few lines, and then give myself the luxury of letting my mind drift. From this process come ideas for speeches or columns. It's also one way I get ready for my day.

From my vantage point, I observe the line of people waiting to purchase pastries, bagels, and of course, their Morning Joe. I am intrigued by the tide of patrons; why are they here? What brought each of them? What do they do?

One can immediately tell the vocation of some by their apparel. Health care professionals are adorned in "scrubs." Although of various colors, or decorated with animals, at a glance one can deduce, "She works at a doctor's office."

Of course, public safety employees; fire, law enforcement, ambulance; are easy to ascertain, as is a well-groomed individual in a grey, pin striped suit: "Business Person."

Some of what we do is obvious.

So it was apparent that the thin man in the big-pocketed white jeans with the T-shirt spotted with colors was a painter. Although not a purchased-from-the-rack uniform, his attire – as clearly as a stethoscope declares, "doctor" or dress whites labels a sailor – broadcast his profession.

Some of what we do is obvious.

"I like your column," he said. "I read it all the time."

Setting down my newspaper, I replied, "Thank you." And noticing his size, added, "You don't look like you need to lose weight – or you've been very successful."

He laughed, "No, I don't need to. But I find it inspirational."

I guess it goes without saying that he was friendly (and had good taste, obviously). Our banter meandered politely through the fields of family and weight loss, culminating when he joked about now being embarrassed because he was buying a donut. Waving and smiling as the glass door swung into place behind him, he left the bakery and was absorbed in the faceless river of people racing to work. My attitude, a tad dour when I entered the business, had brightened. I found myself smiling.

Some of what we do is obvious. Some – not so much.

Sometimes, a trivial act, a kind simple gesture can – even without conscious realization – uplift another. A stranger's comments such as the painter to me; or holding open a door for a stranger; complimenting a co-worker, "Nice blouse;" any of these can change the face of another's day. We don't know it will, because it's "just something we do." But it surely does.

So too does taking care of oneself. Too often, we mistakenly believe we're making it difficult for those around us as we become conscious of our choices and alter our patterns. But, reality is they look at us as an inspiration, satisfied that someone they love is taking better care of herself. They feel proud, sharing our joy.

We might not see that, certainly not at first. But watching over our health also uplifts our family and friends. Like the ripple caused by a stone thrown into a lake it reaches shores we might not see.

The painter inspired me. Hopefully, I have passed forward. Give it to someone else.

He probably thought he was just being friendly, but it didn't make it any less valuable.

Some of what we do is obvious. Some – not so much. Do it anyway.

CAN WE LEGISLATE BEAUTY?

Deborah Rhode, a Stanford law professor, recently published "The Beauty Bias: The Injustice of Appearance in Life and Work." In her book, she puts forth the argument that appearance-based discrimination is pervasive. She also proposed that it could be addressed, at least in part, through legislation, in effect, "anti-lookism" laws. Her conclusions flow from the reality that employees report looks-based discrimination at about the same rate as gender or racial discrimination and that such unfairness translates into loads of other tangible problems.

This is not a novel concept; six cities and one state already forbid various kinds of appearance-based discrimination. Michigan outlawed height and weight discrimination in the 1970s. The city of Santa Cruz bans discrimination based on any physical characteristic outside the individual's control. (No one has ever filed a complaint in the 15 years the law has been on Santa Cruz's books and Michigan sees about 30 complaints and one lawsuit a year due to its law.)

I learned of Ms. Rhode's ideas while reading a Newsweek column by Dahlia Lithwick. Ms Lithwick points out, "discrimination against unattractive women and short men is as pernicious and widespread as bias based on race, sex, age, ethnicity, religion, and disability." She cites an ice-water-in-your-face statistic: "Eleven percent of surveyed couples say they would abort a fetus predisposed toward obesity. College students tell surveyors they'd rather have a spouse who is an embezzler, drug user, or a shoplifter than one who is obese."

Let's rewind: Eleven percent would get an abortion if they felt their unborn child was pre-disposed to obesity?! College couples would rather have a criminal for a life-partner instead of someone who is obese??! I am shocked and saddened; not from some naïve belief that looks matter not but because of how much emphasis we put on one's external attributes, instead of what really matters, what resides inside.

In many ways, we have progressed. Boorish comments about race, heritage, gender, ability, and intelligence are looked at with disgust. The purveyor of such statements is often isolated and shunned. Yet – in many places – a churlish remark about one's physical characteristics is still considered up to standard, even witty.

Even if I thought legislation was the right approach to cure such societal ills, how could it be enforced? Will we post beauty cops at street corners? Will some futuristic mega-attractive society require us to have our Body Mass Index tested as regularly as our driver's license?

Yet, it begs a much deeper question. What is "beauty?"

A celebrity supermodel who will not control her rage and hurls objects at her employees is far more unsightly than a plump receptionist with what I might consider to be a poorly designed hairstyle and an unfortunate choice of outfits. Is a well-toned athlete with a foul temper and a pattern of cheating on his spouse more appealing to us than a rotund, undersized, middle-aged fellow who dotes on this family and brings an uplifting sense of humor to his workplace? I sense not.

I do not think we can legislate such opinions, but the very conversation of whether or not we can or should calls for us to re-evaluate yet again which traits we deem as appealing. Speaking for myself, I know short men to whom I must look up. And I am fortunate to know heavy women who lighten my life.

Brittany's first steps

Dinner had finished so they retired to the living room, leaving the pile of plates and cups in the sink. After all, dishes will wait, your daughter's potential first steps will not.

Brittany, a curly-haired, energetic, bundle of energy; was their only child. In her ten months on this planet, she was a never-ending source of exploration, undaunted and undeterred by any obstacle (causing mom and dad to have quick reflexes on more than one occasion). Tonight would hopefully be "the night." So, Randy and Teresa patiently watched as Brittany crawled along the brown thick carpet from couch to love seat and back again.

Upon arriving at each target, she would pull herself to a standing position, waver unsurely for a moment (always glancing for approval to mom and dad), and then either inadvertently flop down hard on her diaper-clad bottom, or collapse back to the floor on to her hands and knees, crawling on to the next locale, repeating the process. As Randy told anyone who asked (and many who didn't), "She was ready to evolve from a horizontal noise unit to a vertical one." To prepare for the auspicious event, the house was at the ready; all breakables were relocated, electric sockets were covered, and the digital camera was always nearby.

All that remained was for the star to make her grand entrance.

Brittany let go of the couch, outstretched chubby arms toward Teresa, who snapped up the camera.

"Randy," she called, "This is it!"

"Yeah, I see!" He flipped the switch on the camcorder and the red LED glowed under the lens.

"Come on sweetie," Teresa said, holding out her hand to welcome Brittany in her direction. "You can do it."

"Look at daddy's big girl," added Randy. "Come on Honey!"

A slobbering smile, adorned with four white teeth, crossed her face as she let go of the sofa cushion and wobbled like an infant Frankenstein's monster toward mommy, who was snapping photos as quickly as the batteries would recharge. Dad, low on the ground, trying for an artistic "POV," let the video roll. The budget might have been small, but the scene had all the excitement of any Hollywood blockbuster.

Brittany continued to place one chubby foot in front of the other, staggering ever forward. She took a rickety second step, followed by a shaky third. Losing equilibrium on her fourth, she collapsed on to her bottom and exploded in surprised giggles while she clapped for herself.

Teresa and Randy bolted toward their daughter, joining in the celebration. Scooping her up, overflowing with as much joy and pride as if the little one won an Academy Award, Teresa hugged Brittany tightly and began spinning with her in circles. Randy danced a quirky jig around the both of them, waving his arms overhead like some form of dancing chimpanzee, chanting, "Who's daddy's walking girl? Brittany's her name! That's right! You got it! Uh-huh, uh-huh!"

Brittany clapped. Everyone laughed. Mom cried (so did Dad, but he tried to hide it) and after a few moments, Brittany indicated she wanted back on the floor. After all, there was walking to be done – and nothing was going to stop her now, certainly not after an enthusiastic reaction like this.

One unsure step, slightly awkward, and definitely unbalanced; but she was on her way, one tiny foot in front of the other. She would fall. She would get up again. At times, she might not even know where she was headed, but she knew she'd get there. She just had to keep moving.

THE PAIN AND BENEFITS OF CHANGE

Jute is a long, soft, shiny vegetable fiber that can be spun into coarse, strong threads. Produced from plants in the genus Corchorus, family Tiliaceae, it is second only to cotton in amount produced and variety of uses.

I bet you didn't know that, huh?

Of course, the composition of my yoga mat is nowhere near top of consciousness as I glare point blank at it while my schnoz hovers a few inches over it. I am frantically trying to quell the screaming in my deltoids while attempting to discover inner peace engaged in "Dolphin pose," in my Yoga class.

To experience this posture, stand with feet parallel. Then bend forward from the waist so your elbows rest on your mat in front of you. Then interlock your fingers into a fist. The final pose will look like a triangle whereby the top half of your body forms one side, your protruding hindquarters and legs form a second, and the floor becomes the third. Dolphin pose also provides you a macro view of all the grime on the floor while providing the additional benefit of placing your nose barely inches above it.

However, as they say in late night TV commercials, "But wait! There's more!"

Once your Achilles tendon is stretched beyond what you thought was humanly possible, and you are supporting the entire weight of your upper body on bony, aching elbows, glide forward and backward so your noggin slides from the tip of your interlocked fingers back to your elbows. Do not place your knees on the ground, but make sure your heels are.

To imagine the full effect, picture the pain of attempting too many push-ups with the strain of too many pull-ups. Now, just for kicks and giggles, throw in that aching feeling you get in your shoulders after crouching over a computer all day. This is all available to you in only seconds, rather than hours.

Ah, the refreshing feeling of Yoga!

So, there I am as my Yoga instructor reminds me to breathe in, letting my Prana, life force, fill me. I cannot speak for others, but my life force is thinking of a hot shower and a soft bed.

That's when it happened. I won't lie and say the pain vanished. It didn't – on no, not by a long shot. However, after attending Yoga classes for almost a year, something snapped (um, poor choice of words); something changed and, for an instant, I found myself in a mental place where, although I could feel discomfort, I also experienced exhilaration because, until this moment, I was never before able to achieve this pose. (Why I would want to is a question to remain unanswered for now.) Excitement flooded my soul; I pushed myself further.

It occurred to me that – should I have stopped taking my classes at six months, or three, or one – I would never have experienced this level of accomplishment; this serenity. One inch. One class. One more day.

Isn't that change? We get so locked up trying to avoid its pain that we overlook its benefits. We give up, stagnant, overwhelmed, defeated. Change is discomfort, yes, but sticking with it also provides a sense of peace, pride, and accomplishment. As they say, "Don't quit five minutes before the miracle happens."

All that said, I admit I still look forward to "Corpse pose," the relaxation posture at the end of session. The name explains how it looks.

ON THE (BUTTER)
HORNS OF A DILEMMA

Here I sit, having facetime with the perennial decision of any dieter, "Do I or don't I?"

Somebody said that foods made with salt, sugar, and fat are the most irresistible. Why not just call them what they are, "baked goods?" I am practically captive to their doughy gooey pull; Homer strapped to the mast, whilst the sweet scent of glaze sings upon the wind unto me. If not for the pull of the ropes of self-restraint, I would fall victim to their fetching, alluring, siren-quality magnetism, throwing myself full-force into a mound of éclairs, finding light only after munching and devouring my way to the top.

Yet, when rational thought surfaces, I am aware that the self-control now under assault is the ground floor of everything I have accomplished. My head is held higher, my stomach is flatter, my blood pressure is lower, my muscles are tighter. By no coincidence, these all exist in the same period when my self-esteem is Everest high.

I am no Johnny-come-lately to healthful eating, recognizing that a weight gain is neither the result of ONE bear claw nor a SOLITARY cake donut with extra sprinkles. Conversely, I am also weary; as the precipitous journey begins with a single, minor step. The rapid slide from grace is birthed by a thoughtless, momentary, loss of control. It is not food itself that causes obesity; rather one's midsection expands due to an infection of the thoughts: "There's always tomorrow," or, "Just this once," or "What's the use?"

On some wondrous occasions, my thoughts are ill equipped to ver-balize how adrenalized am I about taking care of myself. At once, I am excited, enthused, motivated, energized, inspired, happy, radi-ant and effusive; just to scratch the surface. I proclaim broadly my successes to anyone within earshot. I post it on my blog and send it worldwide via email. Should four commuters be waiting at a bus stop, they become fair game to hear my testimony of success. Life is grand. All is at it should be.

Yet…

There are those "other" moments when I would rather endure a root canal sans Novocain than spend one more second monitoring fat and fiber grams, calculating calories, weighing portions, track-ing food intake, and reading labels. I have had my fill of conscious eating, healthy thinking, and positive affirmations. Should yet one more unexpecting soul make the well-intentioned mistake of re-minding me, "Nothing tastes as good as thin feels," it is not outside the scope of reality that I might lose control and silence such drivel by forcefully shoving full his blathering pie hole with three gallons of rocky-road, peanut brickle, high-fat ice cream. In those times, I cannot be counted as reasonable. But part of being human is to know we all go through them. Anyone who tells you he doesn't is either criminally oblivious or a liar.

This is the yin and yang, ebb and flow, push and pull of dieting; joy and frustration each swirling about, chomping at the bit to make known their presence at any moment. They coexist without end; to make one rise or the other fall, we merely change focus. And the nice thing is, that is always within my power.

Changing the view

I stood on my head today. Well, that's not exactly accurate. Actually standing on my head would require a level of flexibility and dexterity not possessed by yours truly as my feet cannot even reach that big ol' noggin of mine. Besides, even if they could, why would I choose to stand on it? It would be painful, and I would get footprints on my ears.

So, I guess the more precise way to describe it is, "I did a headstand." Really! There I was: head where my feet usually are and feet where my head goes (except when sleeping of course).

I found myself in this most topsy-turvy world because my Yoga teacher says it is beneficial as it helps with blood pressure and reduces stress (well, except for your arms; they were stressed quite the big amount, let me tell you). Since I started Yoga, she has been urging, guiding, cajoling, and coaxing to get me to try this top-is-bottom bizarre configuration.

I get pleasure from Yoga; and the more I'm doing it, the more I appreciate that it's not about turning oneself into a human pretzel. There is extreme satisfaction from enhanced flexibility, increased strength, and better posture. Add to that, that I can now bend down (and get back up) without a written plan, and that I have enhanced my spirituality; and it's gosh-darn difficult to come up with reasons why I would limit myself. However, when my teacher gets that "we're-going-to-go-upside-down" twinkle in her eye, I freak out. The way I see it is if God wanted us to be downside up, he would have put hats on our feet and shoes on our ears.

OK, the actuality is doing something this different from my norm is just plain frightening. There, I've said it! The fear is further amplified because all my inner talk reminds me of everything that could go askew. Of course, I was scared that I would look stupid – or worse yet, what happens if I fall down and get hurt? Valid concerns, sure, but I'll come clean: the genuine bottom line (or would it be "top line" in this case?) is that I lacked faith in myself and was sure I would fail. I can be my own worst limitation.

So, as I lowered my face to the floor in modified dolphin pose, she said, "Breathe out the fear. Relax your shoulders. Raise your strong leg…"

I lifted it. I breathed.

"Make it tight. Pull to the midline."

She assisted by supporting my outstretched leg.

"Now, lift your other leg."

So, I exhaled, lifted it, pulled to my midline, and before I could say, "I can't do this," I did. There I was; head in hands, feet on the wall; vertical – and flabbergasted at what I could do when I didn't tell myself I couldn't. Like most of life, it took some assistance, a tad of discomfort, and a bit of faith. Yet the benefits linger beyond the act.

I feel like – no, I take that back – I AM a new person now. I recognize it's just a Yoga pose; I didn't change the world or cure cancer; but I am holding my head up higher now (in more ways than one), and carrying myself with enhanced confidence. As a matter of fact, the whole world looks different today, more colorful, alive, and brighter.

One could say I began seeing things from a whole new point of view.

WHAT REALLY MATTERS

Despite my jeremiad about the barbarian state of airline travel, one upside of "professional speaker-dom" is that I attend conventions where the speakers are – at the risk of being a cheerleader for my vocation – pretty darn good. However, the pinnacle of any homily I have ever delivered from the platform was but an anthill in comparison to one of the most compelling, powerful presentations I have ever had the good fortune to listen to while at the annual National Speakers Association gathering.

In an ordeal you might remember, Nando Parrado and his soccer teammates, endured more than two tortuous months stranded in the snow-covered Andes 14,000 feet above sea level at temperatures dropping to negative 40 degrees. He, with his teenage teammates, sister, and mother, was flying from Uruguay to Argentina to compete in a weekend soccer excursion. All were to return home the following Monday.

Events did not unfold as expected.

Off-course more than 100 miles, their airplane – after slamming at full force into the top of a mountain – snapped into two, lost its wings, impacted another peak, and – after all that – slid hell-bent at triple-digit speed down a glacier; until finally coming to an unforgiving, more-than-abrupt termination because it slammed full speed into a rocky outgrowth. The cockpit was crushed; the pilots were killed. Of the 46 on board, 29 miraculously survived, only to endure one of the most unbearable – and at the same time, marvelous – testaments to human perseverance ever recorded.

Left with a transistor radio, one package of peanuts, and one chocolate bar to sustain those who did not perish, they took what limited shelter they could in the busted, shattered wreckage of the torn remnants of the fuselage. Two weeks after impact, adding a hellish insult to this nightmare, several more survivors were killed when the mountain unleashed an avalanche, burying the troop under twelve feet of snow.

After two months, unable to "take it any more," and losing all hope of rescue, Parrado and a teammate – adorned merely in jeans, T-shirts, and make-shift shoe shoes – trekked, hiked, crawled, and dragged themselves 70 miles down the mountain, eventually finding help, and rescuing the 16 remaining survivors. (His mother and sister did not make it.)

"I am not a hero," he recalled, his words scented with the slight aroma of a Latin accent, "I was a teenage boy. I simply wanted to survive."

"Today, I am not bothered by what others call problems. Compared to those times on top of the mountain, I have no problems," he said, "Sometimes, I merely have a few 'issues.'"

"My greatest lesson was not how to survive, but rather what is significant in life: those we love. Every day," he reminded us, "Tell those important to you how you feel. We think they will be waiting for us at day's end. But that will not always be the case. Never pass on an opportunity to focus on what really matters, people."

As his talk ended, the lights came up, and the longest standing ovation I have ever witnessed quieted; we speakers, silently exited the expansive ballroom, returning to our conference schedule of hallway meetings, seminars, and breakout sessions; no one ashamed of the red rings around their eyes.

I know I was not the only person who pulled from its holster a cell phone. I tapped into it my wife's number, and left a message telling her how much I love her and what a blessing she is in my life.

I did it again today. I will do it tomorrow, and every day until I can no more.

LESSONS FROM A CHILD

She was dressed in pink sweatpants with the word, "sweet" emblazoned on her diaper-clad bottom. On her feet were brown clogs. Atop her head was a wool, knitted, patchwork cap of pink, yellow, and red, giving her a pastel "Rastafarian" look. However, instead of dreadlocks wrapped within, a waterfall of blonde, bouncy, curls framed her wide-open blue eyes and light complexion.

In her chubby, small, right hand, she carried what used to be a cookie; now, however, all that remained was a half eaten, saliva-covered, dollop of doughy goo with a smattering of pink frosting encrusting the edges. "Cookie" in hand, she bounded as if on springs from one corner of the bakery to the other, her grandfather always in eye shot, as she pointed to each of the items on the bottom shelf of the bakery's glass case, looking to him for the correct word.

"Cookie," he said, as she pointed to a green, sprinkle covered cutout of a dinosaur.

She inspected the pastry, decided she was satisfied with his answer, and then proceeded to the next item, pointing her finger at the glass and looking to him for the mot juste.

"Donut," he said.

"Dunt," she echoed.

"Yes, that's right: donut," he replied, smiling and tussling her cap.

As she progressed along the casing, "bagel," "bearclaw," and "éclair" were added to her lexicon.

As young ones are prone to do, she became bored with the vocabulary lessons and resumed her exploration of the room, lifting and rising with each alternate footfall, swinging her gooey mass of drooly cookie remnant in her right hand. Methodically, she approached – one by one – the patrons at each table; each of whom couldn't help but smile (and this one in particular who was inspired by her actions to write).

As she made eye contact with each of us, there was no fear of judgment in her expression; no self-doubt, questioning what others thought of her actions. In this moment, at this time, she was complete, everything she needed to be. All in her world was perfect.

They – whomever "they" are – have erroneously told us that confidence is acquired as the result of years on the planet. Yet, after observing this energetic, welcoming, unabashed toddler, I wonder; maybe self-assurance is our birthright – not the self-doubt with which we saddle ourselves. As we grow older, in many ways we have become less ourselves, not more; little by little giving up what we want for fear of what "they" might say. And therefore, we put off our goals, we hide our dreams under a bushel, and rarely do we rise to the glory of who we can be. Said nineteenth century British politician, Benjamin Disraeli, "Most people will go to their graves with their music still in them."

Her adventure in the bakery now complete, a small white paper bag now clutched in her fist where the mushy pastry had been, she left the business, waving "bye-bye" to each of the customers while her grandfather held patiently open the heavy glass door.

It's interesting how much you can pick up from someone who can't even speak a word.

I THINK THEREFORE I BECOME

Next to my bed is a nightstand. I presume that is a common arrangement in many bedrooms. Upon the shelf of the nightstand are many books; this too I assume is widespread. Like me, I take for granted that many people have three categories of books populating their nightstands:

Some wait to be read. While at a bookstore, the concept between its covers was so striking that I plunked down money, thinking, "I will read that someday." Alas, "someday" has yet to make its appearance. Being optimistic, I'm sure it will (probably about the same time as when "I get my act together").

The second classification is books started but still unfinished. Maybe I lost interest, the story was not as expected, or simply "life kicked in." I could give them away but feel like I betrayed them, (does co-dependence apply to books?) so I pledge to finish reading them in the future. Until that fateful moment, they too shall gather dust.

Finally comes the definitive category: Books completed. Residing here include authors such as Robert B. Parker, Dean Koonz, and Roger McBride Allen. Most are novels because I like to "escape." However, there is one self-help book I have read over and over again. Although I do not buy into everything she says, *How To Heal Your Life* by Louise Hay is infused with 210 pages of brilliantly simple wisdom (usually the best kind).

Hay's philosophy, outlined in the foreword, includes:

- We are each responsible for our experiences
- Resentment, criticism, and guilt are damaging, and
- It's only a thought, which can be changed.

Furthermore, says Hay, feelings are "thoughts that stick."

This begets clarification. Most of our stream of consciousness flowing between our ears is emotionally neutral. However, periodically, for better or worse, we draw a thought from the current and focus on it. The longer we drill, the more emotional the thought. Emotions drive change. Change affects our future. So, put two and two together and one can see that thoughts actually do manifest themselves as our lives.

For example, I weigh 179 pounds. This is a statement of fact, a thought that might fire across my synapses upon stepping on a scale. It is as colorless as mayonnaise on white bread. However, should I place deep attention upon it, I might generate follow-up thoughts such as, "Is 179 a good weight or a bad weight? … What do others weigh? … How come some weigh less? … Should I weigh less also? … Why don't I weigh what they weigh? … I must not be as good as they are."

Voila! From a neutral thought is born an emotion; in this case, a negative, limiting sentiment comparing myself unfavorably to others and placing myself in a position of inferiority. I have now made myself feel bad, incapable, damaged. Because of that, I am inclined to spend my time lurking in emotionally dark places, less disposed to attempt new things, maintaining the status quo – and most likely consoling myself with copious amounts of chocolate.

Conversely, should I determine 179 is a mighty fine number, thank you very much; one of which I feel proud; I am empowered, energized, and uplifted. I pursue life with fervor and engage it readily, all from a position of strength.

The thought, the number, is neutral. What words I use in my internal dialogue about it decide my feelings. Should I feel unhappy, stagnant, or trapped; it might be a beacon that it's time to change my thoughts; an idea certainly worth thinking about.

ATTENDING HIS
FIRST MEETING

"So, I just went to my first meeting. I thought I'd call and let you know."

I was eager to hear about it but didn't want to come across as "too" eager; might scare him from talking. "I'm proud of you. How are you doing?"

Brief pause, analyzing his feelings; "Hard to explain, really. I felt extremely awkward when I first walked in. I really wanted to turn and run, but I decided I came this far; I'll stay until I feel comfortable."

"And did you get more comfortable?"

"Not much. I guess I've got to keep going back until I do."

"Great attitude," I said. "I can only imagine how much courage it took to show up. We've been talking about it for years. What made you finally decide to go?"

"I realized things weren't going to get any better until I made them better. I'm tired of feeling bad all the time. I felt like I was trapped. I was always angry. I was ruining my relationships. It was just time. Any of the above; all of the above, you name it."

"I'm glad you decided to take care of yourself."

"Yeah, I know it's going to be a long journey but I might as well get started. It's not going to get any shorter by waiting, is it?"

I chuckled, "No, you're probably right. So, can you tell me what it was like?"

"Well, there were about 30 people, about five of us were first-timers. I introduced myself when they asked who was new. Everyone said, 'hi,' just like you see in the movies. Then, several people got up and told stories. I sat and listened."

"Hear anything useful?"

"Yeah, several people sounded like they were telling my story, always trying to do everything perfect, getting really upset when other people don't do what they say, blaming everyone else for what goes wrong; you know how I can get."

"Yes I do."

"One guy talked about the difference between peace and serenity. He used a grocery store example. Want to hear it?"

"Sure, I really would."

"He said, 'You know when you stand in line at the checkout and the sign says MAXIMUM 10 ITEMS? You've achieved peace when you see someone in front of you with 12 items and you don't let it bother you.'"

"How do you know when you've achieved serenity?"

"When you don't count the items."

"I like that."

"Me too. I'm tired of counting everyone's items. I've got to take care of my own if I want things to get better."

"How did everyone treat you?"

"Really warm; very, very friendly. Nobody knew me. But they didn't care. They all seemed really glad to see me, shook my hand, welcomed me to the meeting. I felt like I was coming home to family. That's part of the reason I'll go back."

"So, I know it's only your first meeting, but did you hear anything special?"

"Oh yeah, I've got loads to think about."

"What stands out?"

Long pause, "Nothing happens until you ask for help. There are lots of people who will help, but you've got to open the door."

EAT LESS; EXTEND YOUR LIFE

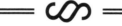

There is no more sought-after dream than that of eternal life.

Since Ponce de Leon set foot in the new world – and well before that – we have been seeking the fountain of youth, the ability to live longer in good health. "We're so close to adding another 20 to 50 years to the human lifespan, that not only are we in the neighborhood, we're on the block; we're just looking for the right door," I was recently informed. The key to the house remains hidden.

For yeast, flies, and rodents however, it's time to party! Scientists have long known that dramatically cutting calories extends their lives. (Who knew that yeast even ate?) Alas, since we do not cavort among baking additives, we have been left out of such advances. Yet, there is hope.

In a recent report, it was discovered that rhesus monkeys, arguably more our kin than yeast, that have been put on a low-calorie diet live longer and healthier lives. Researchers divided 38 monkeys into two groups. One group was put on a diet with 30 percent fewer calories than the other. After two decades, five of the monkeys on the restricted diet had died of normal age-related causes, compared with 14 monkeys on the normal diet. Beyond that, the monkeys on the restricted diet were healthier overall, with no diabetes, and fewer cases of cancer or cardiovascular disease.

"The monkeys on a normal diet also looked visibly older, their eyes more sunken in and their coats thinner and posture cramped when compared with their dieting counterparts," according to Ricki J. Colman, lead author of the paper.

It is assumed that since monkeys and humans are genetic cousins, such diets might slow aging in people, too. However, due to the long lifespan of people and the rigors of the diet, studies of calorie restriction in humans are ongoing and have yet to show that people live longer. Nonetheless, thousands of individuals now follow calorie restriction diets, hoping to discover what de Leon did not.

In the interest of understanding what life would be like on a calorie-restricted diet, I did some research and found a typical "day in the life." Here, soup to nuts, is the purported menu required for a longer time on this planet.

Breakfast: one cup nonfat cottage cheese, 23 nuts, one cup berries, one nutrition bar

Lunch: five ounces skinless chicken breast (boiled, baked or roasted), broccoli, cauliflower, one tablespoon olive oil, one medium orange

Meal preparation: Cook chicken. Add to plate with broccoli and cauliflower. Add olive oil and herbs and spices. Have orange for dessert.

Snack: one cup nonfat yogurt, six nuts (Whoa! Don't eat them all in one bite!)

Dinner: Two cups green, leafy salad (may include lettuce, cabbage, spinach), three ounce salmon filet (canned low-salt or fresh-baked), seven ounce sweet potato (baked), one tablespoon olive oil, herbs and spices, one tablespoon vinegar

Meal preparation: Sprinkle vinegar, herbs, spices and half of olive oil over salad and salmon. Sprinkle remaining olive oil over sweet potato; have potato for dessert.

There you have it, the bill of fare to achieve a longer life. Don't get me wrong; I plan on hanging out on Mother Earth for many a decade. However, if a sweet potato smattered with a few drops of oil for dessert is the price to live to 125, I'm not quite sure it's worth it. Maybe I could have a chocolate bar once in awhile and make it to 120.

An effort either way

From the moment she entered the jet, I could tell she did not want to be there. In addition to apologizing each time her overloaded "Big Brown Bag" banged someone in an aisle seat, she was having difficulty navigating her excessive size down the skeletal-sized aisle.

I knew the other passengers were thinking, "I hope she doesn't sit next to me." Plane seats are not known for roominess, and having someone else's bulk overspill into one's limited area was not something for which anyone eagerly plunked down a few hundred dollars.

My overweight past flooded to my forethought and I remembered being the recipient of "that look" in the other passengers' eyes when I used to enter an airplane. I avoided eye contact; my method of signaling to each traveler, "Don't worry. You're safe. I'm not sitting next to you."

Finally, I would locate my seat (God forbid it was a center seat). I'd smile and meekly point to the location into which I was supposed to compress. My neighbor would smile weakly, rise, and let me pass. After I settled in, he would reclaim his territory and – although he would usually try to hide it – I would notice a subtle, but definite, slight tilt in the opposite direction from me; trying to retain as much space as possible for himself.

All of those memories swamped my consciousness now and I knew what this woman walking the aisle was experiencing in this moment.

As embarrassed as I am to admit it, I felt ashamed because – despite my empathy – I too was hoping her seat assignment would not be next to mine. Realizing with horror what I was thinking, I wanted to spare her "the look" coming from one who had been there, so I pulled up the airline magazine and pretended to be engrossed with two Smiling Solar Tiki Garden Torches that will "light up my corner of paradise."

Eventually she dropped her heft into the seat across the aisle, and shyly lifted her hand to signal the attendant. I also understood that motion; it was code for "I need a seatbelt extension," one more humiliation in an already degrading experience.

"Uncomfortable" would not be a word that even came close to describing the pained expression etched on her face after she was finally able to lift her midsection and insert the tab into the buckle. She was sweating from the exertion of what, to most, is a simple task. Her efforts to normalize her breathing were complicated by the tightness of the belt, the metal stabbing arms of the seat on either side, and, of course, the infamous lack of legroom – made even worse by the baggage she could barely insert under the seat in front of her. It was beyond obvious that she would rather be anywhere but in that spot at that time in this moment.

I really know nothing about the lady on the plane; possibly she was already down several pounds on a diet – or she wasn't. I cannot know; more importantly, it is not my job to judge. But, what I cannot deny is watching her made my heart hurt because it brought back my own experiences. That's an important reminder.

Sometimes, in the effort to improve, I think we get sidetracked, complaining about the effort. "It's too hard." "It'll take too long." We lament the process instead of celebrate our growing freedoms.

Watching her try to relax on a noisy, overcrowded, restrictive airplane in a cramped seat with an overstretched seat belt strangling her midsection reminded me how much better I feel when I take care of myself. Sure, it takes work. Yes, it can be uncomfortable. But, it's a heck of a lot less uncomfortable than doing nothing.

RULES FOR BEING HUMAN

My email spam blocking system informs me that I have received 128,747 email messages of which 68.05 percent were spam. Why I would want to know those particular factoids eludes me. Yet there they reside, utilizing several of my already overworked synapses.

However, what my spam-catching system cannot tell me is how many of my 41,134 approved messages were forwarded, usually commencing, "I normally don't forward things like this but…"

Upon opening said missive, I am informed that Bill Gates will send me $5,000 if I pass this along; or am reminded of the navy ship telling the lighthouse to move; or – more likely – a friend is warning me that if I don't forward this, I shall suffer severe tragedies. (Point of interest: What kind of "friend" would send me something as horrific as that? Just wondering…)

And as long as I got me started, two notes about e-forwarding "etiquette."

One: If you absolutely INSIST on doing it, do not – repeat DO NOT – include all the other comments from everyone and their brother. No one wants to scroll through 67 pages of ">>You gotta see this…" or ">>Send to everyone you know." Delete others' comments; send what matters – but only if necessary, please.

Number Two: If you wish to respond, use REPLY, not REPLY ALL.

Jeeze! They oughta take that button away from people who don't know how to use it. The only thing worse than 67 pages of comments is 67 emails replying with, "COOL," or "BITCHEN, THANKS!"

Oops, excuse the tirade; pet peeve; I got sidetracked. Now, where was I?

Oh yes, once in a while, something great does cross my computer screen, and it's worth telling others about. The RULES FOR BEING HUMAN, by Cherie Carter-Scott, fits that bill, consisting of ten brilliant lessons on how to manage your time on Planet Earth.

They start simply: "You will receive one body. You may like it or hate it, but it will be yours for the entire time you're here." I mean, how much time do we spend glaring at our profile in any passing shiny surface, bemoaning the fact that we don't look like Anglina Jolie or Jennifer Aniston? (Personally, I don't waste a lot of time doing that, but I have unfavorably compared myself to Brad Pitt.) It's not conceit to accept your strong points. Sure, work on our weaknesses. But shame is not attractive so you might as well get rid of it.

The Rules also remind us, "There are no mistakes, only lessons. A lesson will be presented to you in various forms until you learn it. When you have learned it, you can then go on to the next lesson."

How many times have I done the same thing over and over, fooling myself by the preface, "This time it will be different." Sorry, this time will be like the last 17 times, unless I actually do something different.

"Don't you think you might try something else?" asks the

Universe.

"I don't want to," whines my cranky inner kid.

Ultimately, I begrudgingly accept that the Universe will not change it rules to accommodate my whims fantasies or desires and proceed forward. Stomp fee. Kick loudly. Next lesson please.

Altogether, there are ten rules, covering all phases and aspects of existence. Each is simple. All are brilliant. And they end with, "You will forget all these."

You'd think, after all these years in this body, I might understand how things work. You'd think that – but you'd be wrong.

P.S. Please forward this article to everyone on your email list.

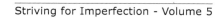

I AM OUTRAGED

Let me jump to the point: I am concerned that we, as a people, are drowning in an epidemic of outrage. Maybe it's not as apparently dangerous as the swine flu, but it is far more virulent and certainly more contagious. It seems that virtually everyone is "outraged" about something or another. We appear to seek out reasons to feel offended, flipping it on as effortlessly as we turn on the hallway light. I am saddened that we are becoming humorless and without joy.

I was prompted into this observation because recently I wrote what I thought was a playful look at fried foods available to me on a trip to New Orleans. I admit to taking license with the details; yet overall, the premise was true: due to the preponderance of deep fried options, I find it harder to stick to my diet in the South. One might even consider it a compliment to southern cuisine. One might, yet, that is not how it was taken. I recently made the mistake of wading into the cesspool of on-line comments posted by some readers. "Outraged" was the main entrée on the menu of insults.

One person pronounced, "The South won't miss your rude and snotty little yankee-on-a-diet attitude," wondering if I was "raised by salad eating wolves," (Huh?) and concluding, "You're real lucky none of those Good Ole Southern Boys heard your pansy **** complaining ... or they would have schooled you on proper etiquette in the Deep South." Ouch. "Bitter, table for one please."

Someone else was enraged I was bringing my "ugly American" attitude where it didn't belong. Isn't New Orleans part of America? I don't know whether to be insulted or confused.

Sussing out a new column, I searched the internet for, "I am outraged." Presented with over one million listings; I entered a virtual culture of enraged, upset, venomous folk; ready to jump onto the seeing red bandwagon at the drop of a hat. Outrage boiled over because of the approval of an artificial sweetener by the FDA. Indignation was rampant because a baseball player opted for elbow surgery. There was high dudgeon because Queen Frostine, a character in the game Candyland, had been demoted to Princess. So distressed was he by such discrimination, that he made a solemn pledge to never again buy another game from the manufacturer, and was arranging a boycott. All is far from sweet in Candyland.

People, please, can we take a breath? Let's slow down long enough to step back from the brink and move distant from the precipice of righteous anger. Let's put the "go-ahead-cross-this-line" bravado on the back burner long enough to hear what someone has to say before we puff up, poke our finger in his chest, and give him the piece of mind we think he deserves?

Sure, there are concerns a plenty; enough to last for generations. We face a heating environment, a teetering economic platform, and a divided political system. There are injustices galore on which we can focus. And maybe that's the reason we're so easily thrown into a tizzy at the slightest affront. However, do we have to react like moths to light with "outrage?" How helpful or pleasant is it to live in a 24-hour state of hypertension, tight jaws, and clenched fists?

Maybe – just a thought here – we could try smiling quicker, listening longer, and thinking deeper. It might not help, but it sure couldn't hurt. Of course, if you disagree, I'm sure I'll get outraged letters.

Not as it seems

To say a continental breakfast is simple, is tantamount to saying fire is hot. No duh. Depending on where you spend the night, this mainstay of hotels and motels might present you with coffee, tea, assorted juices, rolls, yogurt, bagels, pastries, and cereal. Periodically, its menu might include sausage, pancakes, or pre-portioned cups of waffle batter and a waffle maker in which to cook it. (Point of interest: They are called "continental breakfasts" because they are the breakfast of choice on The Continent, also known as Europe.)

If it's going to be a while before your next meal however, be wary of the ubiquitous continental breakfast because the primary food-stuffs served in these breakfasts contain a whole lot of empty calories. Count on a rumbling, empty belly and low energy a few hours hence.

So, with that in mind, ever-conscious (some might say "obsessed") with taking care of myself and watching my weight, I walk the aisle of offerings before making my decision, taking a casual glance at what is available. Too many calories and too much fat in sausage; too much sugar in the waffles; not in the mood for a mushy apple; what to do?

At the end of the line up, the inn has two dispensing machines that provide two different types of cold cereal. In the front of each dispenser, there is a picture of the box from which they come. I presume they do this so you can tell which cereal is which. However, at first blush, the decision to the health-conscious appears obvious. Note use of the word, "appears."

The same company manufactures both products; yet the similarity ends there. One bin is full of red, yellow, blue, and purple loops caked in sugar. Its container, emblazoned with a loud, cartoonish font, is decked out with a caricature of a varicolored, large-billed bird from Central America, who with gleeful abandon is devouring a bowl of the fruity rings.

The other container, I presume is opting to appeal to the "more mature" morning diner as it consists of a multigrain granola with chunks of assorted nuts and raisins. Its package cover is more demure, adorned with a wholesome, unrefined, typeface; and instead of a cartoon character, there is an enlarged photograph of a spoonful of the salubrious mixture, showing detail of its nourishing goodness. Across the top of the box, above the brand, it boldly proclaims, "Low Fat."

With credit to the manufacture, nutritional information is clearly printed on the top of each box, and that's what caught my eye. The low fat cereal, had three grams of fat and the sugary cereal had only one.

"Odd," I thought, and inspected further. In addition to more fat, it had 230 calories compared to 110. It had 150 grams of sodium versus 135, and it had 18 grams of sugar instead of only 12 for the happy bird.

At first blush, the sugary cereal appears to be the healthier alternative. However, years of learning to avoid such items could not be overcome. I opted for a hard-boiled egg.

A COOKIE WON'T HELP

While drinking my morning coffee and reading the newspaper at the local bakery, I watched as the young parents entered the establishment, a small blond girl with huge, round blue eyes, bundled snuggly against the cold wind, was in tow. While her parents stamped their feet on the doormat to restart the circulation in their legs, the lass was pulled, as if by an unseen magnet, to the pink, green, and purple cut-out cookies in the glass case.

She pointed to the pastries on the bottom shelf, secured safely behind the transparent barrier, and looked upwards to mom. "Cookie?" She was few in words but her eyes expressed a dictionary.

"No," said her mom, "Not now. You can have milk if you'd like, but not a cookie."

Undeterred, she continued to stare down her mom, pointer finger pressed tightly against the glass.

"No," her mom repeated. "It's too early."

No change; defiance; a principle was at stake.

Mom squatted, lowering herself to eye level of the toddler. "I'll tell you what. If you're good today, Daddy will bring you back this afternoon and you can get a cookie then. How about that?"

The young girl considered her option, decided it was acceptable and walked away from the glass.

"Interesting how early it starts," I thought. She can barely use words, but already her rewards are provided in the form of sugary goodness. It reminded me of the joke where Johnny, being the rambunctious young lad that he is, is riding his bike full tilt down the driveway, utilizing all the energy and enthusiasm appropriate to a six year old. Approaching a bump too quickly, he loses control of his two-wheeler and tumbles onto the cement.

Strong, but in pain, he picks up the bicycle and hobbles back to the porch, limping slightly from the accident. Mom inspects his damaged knee, assures him that it's minor, and says, "You know what will make it better?"

"No," answers Johnny. "What?"

"A cookie."

Mom reaches into the bear-shaped ceramic jar on the counter and pulls out a large chocolate chip round reward. She hands it to Johnny, who immediately holds it against his bruised knee.

"When will it make stop hurting?" he asks.

Personally, I think it's fine to take pleasure in the taste of food; it's a sense to enjoy. Yet an overhanging question is "Why are we doing it so much?" I do not believe that the only reason to eat is for sustenance or nutrition; but we also must keep that in the forefront. When we look at the shape of our society today (pun loosely intended), it seems to be apparent that we forgot that we eat to live, not the other way around.

When I'm bored, I want to eat. When I'm sad, I eat. When I'm angry – you got it. You know, there are people who, when they're bored, they read a book? When they're sad, they call a friend; and when they're angry, they take a walk. There's a clinical term for that kind of personality: it's called "skinny."

Those habits didn't develop themselves overnight. Somewhere down the line, they learned something different and their actions took a different path, leading to a healthier life. Maybe, – who knows – as a small child, they were told, "If you're really good, Daddy will take you on a bike ride later today."

We might not be children but a bicycle won't care.

MORE THAN BEING POSITIVE

A column in a recent issue of Newsweek magazine has prompted me to think – always a dangerous practice.

The piece, penned by Julia Baird, was entitled "Positively Downbeat," and the basic thesis was that positive thinking was actually making us all more miserable, rather than happier. As evidence, she sites a study from the General Social Survey by economists Betsey Stevenson and Justin Wolfers of Wharton. They found, that despite three decades of economic growth in America (current tumultuous financial climate excepted), men and women are no happier now than they were in the seventies. To further hit home the point, the study found that women in 1972 were, on the average, actually more content than they are now.

Being a devotee of "positive thinking," I was perplexed. How could it be that lighting a candle rather than cursing the darkness would make us more miserable? Intuitively, it made no more sense to me than a study that came out a few years ago, finding that low-calorie foods caused obesity. As in that report, something was obviously askew.

Ms. Baird references another author, Barbara Ehrenreich, who in her book, "Bright-Sided: How Relentless Promotion of Positive Thinking Has Undermined America," calls positive thinking a "mass delusion." Among other ideas, Ms. Ehrenreich argues that the foundation of positive thinking is the belief that you can will anything you like into happening: recovering from cancer, getting a promotion, becoming a millionaire.

It is in that statement that I found a foothold; believe as you wish, one must also accept that the universe will not change its rules to accommodate our whims, fantasies, or desires.

Positive thinking is not blind, naive, magical wishing. I cannot rub a crystal ball, site solemnly my affirmations, and assume that all will go exactly as I foresee. After all, I might fancy Sandra Bullock and myself alone on a tropical, romantic, desert island, while at the same time, her thoughts are, "not in my lifetime buster." I can posit positive until the furrows in my brow are canals, and still move no closer to Ms. Bullock than the DVD I rent from the video store.

Positive thinking does not materialize nirvana for me. What it does is gives me a stake in my own outcomes; so my life becomes mine, for better or worse. Once I accept that I have the wherewithal to direct my actions, I am empowered, not anointed. With the assumption that I am a (mostly) capable sentient being with talents, ideas, and skills; also comes the responsibility of utilizing those gifts to the best of my ability.

An optimistic outlook will not guarantee a life of luxury or ease, it is simply a tool that allows us to deal with events better when they appear difficult and allow us to further enjoy them when they do not. Positive thinking transfers the impetus of action from "out there" to "in here." But if "in here" continually seeks its happiness "out there," it is a void that will never be filled.

LOCUS OF CONTROL

At the very first session I had with my therapist oh so many years ago, the opening question out of my mouth was, "How long will this take?"

Being ever the smart aleck, he replied, "About 50 minutes."

"No," I responded. "How long will it take until I am fixed; you know, healed; normal?"

I am not alone when it comes to asking that question. One of the first items we want checked off our "to do list of change" is a date specific that we can mark on our calendar alerting us to the face that – voila – goal achieved! Like a prisoner sentenced to hard labor, we want to know how long until we are free.

From a logical point of view, the process of getting from "here" to "there" is actually pretty exhilarating. We find out about ourselves. We discover what we're capable of doing. Others compliment and admire us. Life is new; every sunrise provides the option for multiple new adventures, unwrapping more of whom we really are. It would seem that with so much to gain, we would rather linger luxuriously in the progression instead of charge hell-bent for leather to the other side.

So, what's with the big rush?

I'm not naïve, I am more than aware that it takes work and is, at times, prickly; yet most of our goal-driven society touts reflexively, "anything worth having is worth working for." If I want a good marriage, I will work for it. Raising healthy, happy children is certainly an effort at times. Advancing my career and maintaining my house require expending resources. Certainly the best ME possible is a worthy objective, and therefore stands to reason that it also is worth the elbow grease necessary to achieve it.

We might not always be keen on it, but we are not a people afraid of hard work. So that cannot be the reason why the sprint to the finish line. I believe we are in such a hurry to "get there" because we are terrified of waking up with the realization that we have "lost our motivation."

Like the despondent lover, we plead, "Don't go; please stay. I'll be good. What will happen to me if you leave?" If we can arrive at the altar before being jilted by our fickle paramour, everything will be OK.

Being a student of change (aren't we all?), I am enthralled by our choice of words. After all, words reflect our thoughts. Thoughts determine actions. Watch what you say, it could become your life. Therefore, when we say, "I've lost my motivation," it presupposes that motivation is some foreign entity residing in a distant land. Yet, we are the source of our motivation. We gin it up, and we turn it off. We control it; no one else does. Others can inspire us, coerce us, or force us – but motivate? Not so much. (Ever try and "motivate" a lazy teen? Get my point?)

The premier adjustment on the road to stable, long-term change, is to accept that the locus of control – where decisions are made – is internal, not external. Sure, "stuff" happens, and luck (or fate) can be players. Yet, they are bit parts. I own my spotlight. Once I accept that, the only thing in my way is me.

Patriotism and health care

Said a rather dark-sided friend of mine, "Why do you spend so much time writing about health? We all end up the same way in the end. Why fight the inevitable, might as well just enjoy the time we have."

Said I, adjusting rose-colored glasses, "I disagree. None of us know how much time we have, but good health allows us to enjoy it as long as possible."

Came the reply, "Personally, I think good health is merely the state of dying at the slowest possible pace."

Clunk. Ouch. End of bizarre conversation.

That said, in light of all the discussion lately, I've got a thing or two to say about a thing or two about health care. Since my column is not political in nature, I'll attempt to steer clear of that sticky widget. Yet, I'm assuming, no matter one's political leanings, we agree that something is unwell within our health care system.

They say, "Figures don't lie, liars figure." So knowing I could be stepping into an ugly morass, I still wish share a few statistics that I find particularly noteworthy.

According to the 2006 revision of the United Nations World Population Prospects report, for the period 2005-2010, our country ranks 33 when it comes to infant mortality. We are sandwiched between New Caledonia and Croatia.

On the other end of life, from our own CIA's World Factbook, last updated April 2009, our life expectancy is 50th. A child born in the U.S. today will likely be around for 78.1 years. Combine those statistics with the staggering fact that the Organization for Economic Cooperation and Development (a group representing 30 wealthier, industrialized countries) computed that the United States spent $7,290 per capita on health care, ranking it first among the countries studied.

Might just be me, but I don't think we're getting our money's worth.

Whether the solution is public option or private health insurance is not the issue I'm trying to address. Yes, what our government does might indeed affect us for generations far beyond our (hopefully extending) lifespans. Yes, there is much to be corrected.

But, quoting Cassius, "The fault, dear Brutus, is not in our stars, But in ourselves..." It's easy to pronounce and pontificate about what "they" should do, it's quite another little something to step to the platform, roll up our sleeves, and actually take action. Irrespective of legislation regarding "single payer" or "pre-existing conditions," we must each make a difference in our own lives by establishing good health as a higher priority in day-to-day decisions.

This does not mean uproot and rebuild your entire routine, throwing every habit into the waste bin. Make a small stand if that's all you can do but make it now. Opt for less processed food. Lower your sugar intake. Park your car at the far end of the lot. Small steps done regularly have more impact than big steps done intermittently. In other words, it's better to get out and walk around the block – and really do it – than it is to promise to run a mile someday soon but never get around to it.

Find an excuse to act in a healthier fashion. It feels good; it's even patriotic.

A look at Thanksgiving traditions

The most common Thanksgiving holiday traditions are:

- Giving Thanks
- Thanksgiving Day Parade
- Football
- Breaking the wishbone
- Turkey and Trimmings

I am unclear how the genealogy section of About.com determined this; yet intuitively it appears correct. Ever curious (and always looking for content for my column), I wondered how these came to be; so I did some research. I share.

According to historians, the Pilgrims never observed an annual Thanksgiving banquet in autumn. In the year 1621, they did celebrate a feast following their first harvest, but this ceremony was never repeated. (Oddly, most devoutly religious pilgrims of that time did observe a day of thanksgiving, but they did so by fasting.) George Washington was the first president to declare the holiday, in 1789.

In the mid–1800s, many states – but not all – observed a Thanksgiving holiday. During the Civil War, President Lincoln, looking for ways to unite the nation, discussed the subject with poet and editor Sarah J. Hale, who had been lobbying for Thanksgiving to become a national holiday. In 1863 he gave his Thanksgiving Proclamation and declared the last Thursday in November a day of thanksgiving.

Seeking to lengthen the Christmas shopping season, Franklin D. Roosevelt, in 1939, 1940, and 1941, changed Thanksgiving to the third Thursday in November. Finally, amid controversy, Congress passed a joint resolution in 1941 and since that time, Thanksgiving remains on the fourth Thursday of November.

Of course, giving thanks remains the bedrock of the celebration and our country is not alone in that tradition. Other countries with an official Thanksgiving holiday include Argentina, Brazil, Canada, Japan, Korea, Liberia, and Switzerland.

As for football, the first intercollegiate football championship was held on Thanksgiving Day in 1876. Parades started almost a half-century later when, in 1920, Gimbel's Department Store in Philadelphia organized the first one. Many erroneously credit the first parade to Macy's, which actually began in 1924, and of course, continues to this day.

I did not realize that the wishbone had such a long history. Getting the larger section of the wishbone and making a wish upon it dates back to the Etruscans (who lived in northwestern Italy in the first millennium BC). The Romans brought the tradition with them when they conquered England and the English colonists carried the tradition on to America. For those of us who appreciate the derivation of phrases, the term "lucky break," comes from getting the larger piece.

With regards to the choice of turkey for the main course of the meal, blame or credit that to the evolution of our language. In the 1600s, "turkey" was the generic name to describe all fowl. Actually, many historical accounts of that first feast include references to venison, boiled pumpkin, berries, and, maybe even shellfish.

Although food is definitely a means by which we celebrate good fortune, I must note that nowhere is "stuffing oneself until sick" listed as a tradition. Quite the contrary, I would go so far as to say that uncomfortable, pained, hyper-expanded feeling that follows so many Thanksgiving celebrations actually detracts from the appreciative sense of gratitude one would hope to experience. Maybe, that's one tradition we can drop this year.

Therefore, amid friends and family, let us resolve this year to find more reasons to give thanks, more occasions to help those less fortunate than us, and more ways to take better care of ourselves, starting with a wonderful Thanksgiving.

TOTALLY GROSS

When it comes to food prep, no one would mistake me for a gourmet chef. I mean I can find my way around a kitchen, even prepare a nice meal or two if needed; but if my life hung in the balance, I still couldn't tell you the difference between broccoli and Gai-lohn nor when to use a Dutch oven instead of a stock pot. Most times, if a recipe involves more than a quarter turn in a microwave oven, I'm on to something else.

That said, when I do take the time to prepare a meal, I am conscious of how it looks and of course, how healthy it is. So, I was knocked flat-footed by a relatively new phenomenon sweeping across the good ol' U.S. of A. called the "Gross Food Movement."

This trend, supported by websites such as ThisIsWhyYoureFat.com, sports foods such as the Monster Sandwich Pie, which includes half a roast ham and half a roast turkey, a tub of sour cream, a tub of cream cheese, and a full pound of cheddar and Swiss cheeses, all stuffed inside a King's Hawaiian round bread loaf. As near as I can calculate, this "sandwich" tops the scales at around 12,000 calories – enough to fuel the average body for the better part of a week. No need to wait all those days to get your energy needs; in our rush-rush, gotta-have-it-quickly society; you can carb-load to a brand new level and consume everything you need (and a lot of what you don't) in one meal. (Antacids available separately.)

Looking for something to help wind down at the end of a hard day clogging your arteries with Monster Pies? How about the McNuggetini? This festive drink (?) consists of a chocolate milkshake mixed with vodka, rimmed with barbeque sauce, and garnished with half a chicken nugget. "Hey barkeep! Gimme a double will ya?"

Finally, for dessert, how 'bout a Hot Beef Sundae? Yep, mashed potatoes smothered in brown gravy and cheddar cheese, with a cherry tomato on top. Please, no whipped cream, I'm on a diet.

Some might say the Gross Food Movement (if one can even move after eating such foods) is a playful, fun, fat-laden, extremely greasy, hyper-caloric backlash to the "obsession" we have with healthy eating. They might be right.

Others might say that it's just, well, gross.

I know I am about to come across to some as a stick in the mud. That said, maybe it's my upbringing; maybe it's years of watching my weight (or maybe it's just looking at the photos of the concoctions I described); but I find the whole thing to be extremely wasteful and somewhat sad. Don't get me wrong, I am not advocating food police be established or that new laws and regulations be enacted to restrict such culinary catastrophes; I am just expressing an opinion. In a world where half the population is desperately trying to scrape together enough food to make it through the night, our society is so affluent that we have competitive eating contests and recipe books containing Bacon-Wrapped Pigs In A Blanket Wrapped In Bacon.

If someone wants to cook up an Upside Down Mac & Cheese Pizza (a layer of macaroni and cheese sandwiched between two cheese pizzas), I won't stand in the way. But at the same time, especially this time of year, it would be nice to stop by a shelter and help feed those who would be thankful for what we throw away.

INHALING YOUR MEALS

It would be so much simpler to maintain my weight if it wasn't for that darned need to eat. Think of how thin we'd be. Consider how much money we'd save at grocery stores and restaurants. Imagine watching television without those constant fast-food ads. Alas, 'tis not to be – or is it? Science marches on.

Welcome "Le Whif," produced by David Edwards, the Gordon McKay Professor of the Practice of Biomedical Engineering at Harvard's School of Engineering and Applied Sciences. Professor Edwards has invented a method to get past all that pesky cooking and actual consuming of foods, describing Le Whif as "a new way of eating."

Hmmm … ponder with me. How might one add to the eons-old experience of preparing foodstuffs, putting them in one's mouth, and chewing repetitively? The answer is as clear as the nose on your face: breathe your food. Yep, you read that correctly. However, before you try pounding a hamburger and fries into your nostrils, you might want to know a little more.

Says Edwards: "Over the centuries we've been eating smaller and smaller quantities at shorter and shorter intervals. It seemed to us that eating was tending toward breathing, so, with a mix of culinary art and aerosol science, we've helped move eating habits to their logical conclusion. We call it whiffing."

Personally, I don't buy the basic premise. I do agree that we've been eating in shorter and shorter intervals. After all, can't one describe "non-stop" as the ultimate short interval? Yet, if the quantities were getting smaller and smaller, I doubt that we'd be dieting and dieting, and our waistlines would be expanding and expanding.

Nonetheless, Le Whif has surfaced, delivering about 200 milligrams of chocolate per puff, which is less than one calorie. The FAQs on the web-page explain how it could help with dieting, "When you eat a chocolate bar, most of the chocolate passes through your mouth without actually contacting your taste buds. From a taste point of view, most of the choc-olate is not serving you, apart from delivering calories through digestion. By whiffing, the chocolate has no chance to pass through your mouth without falling on your tongue or other surfaces in your mouth. Most of the chocolate you whiff, you taste. If taste is driving you to eat more than you wish to eat, Le Whif can help." Makes sense to me.

The device looks like a cross between a lipstick tube and an Asthma inhaler, and, in addition to chocolate, one may inhale four other fla-vors: mint, raspberry, mango and plain. Of course, all are calorie-free. Personally, I understand why chocolate is in the list; maybe even the oth-ers. However, wouldn't "plain flavored aerosol" just be air? Couldn't I just take a big old deep breath and have a full whiffy meal without paying for it? I see a hole in the business plan.

For example, I envision a future dinner party. Company enters the house, conversations ensue, hugs are shared. After the small talk, the parade into the kitchen begins. Each person pulls out a chair and gathers around the table.

"Oooh! What flavor are we having tonight?" asks an excited guest.

"Plain," comes the reply. "Take a deep breath. Enjoy. And please help yourself to seconds, there's plenty for everyone."

THE GREATEST GIFT OF ALL

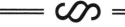

I am one of the underclass of the holiday season – those who wait to the last minute to buy gifts – so I find myself on Christmas Eve in yet another line. The customer at the front; an elderly, bearded, overweight gentleman with thick black heavy boots, and wire rim glasses resting on a pug nose; is having an animated discussion with an apathetic clerk. Shoppers buried under sparkly packages are restlessly shifting from one leg to the other, glancing at watches, and staring at the ceiling as the long-winded debate ricochets back and forth.

The sales person reiterates, "You can't pay for that many toys using pennies."

"That's all I've got. I can't pay you in milk, cookies, or crayon drawings; but sometimes children leave me pennies. That's all I own."

The clerk shrugged. "I'm sorry Sir, you'll have to go elsewhere." He abruptly turns to me, next in line, and disregards the pudgy gentleman.

Trying to avoid looking at the old-timer, but finding it impossible to notice his eyes losing their sparkle, I inform the clerk to charge me for both our purchases. "It is a blessing to give," I tell the shopper as he looks on in amazement.

The heavy man shakes my hand profusely as he lets out a deep robust belly laugh, his middle shaking like jelly, "I'm going to make sure you get something astonishing tomorrow morning! It's my greatest gift!" With that, he again laughed his full, rich, belly-quaking laugh, gathered his packages and hurried into the cold.

The next morning, I raced downstairs, not knowing what to expect – sure that whatever it was, it would be big, or expensive – or both. I surveyed the living room. Nothing. Then the obvious became apparent: "Come on Scott, you're an adult. What were you thinking? How silly to even pretend. He was an eccentric geezer who cashed in his penny jar, that's all." I brushed aside my foolishness and started to exit when I noticed a simple envelope adorned with an embossed snowflake and a monogrammed "S.C." Slitting it open, I pulled out a handwritten note on parchment: "Henceforth, you will realize how fortunate you truly are. Your life is full even when it seems not. Enjoy your blessings. Thanks for the help."

Reverting to my previous analysis of a well-meaning gentleman whose ornaments weren't hanging from the right tree, I shoved the memo into my pocket and cradled a warm cup of tea between my hands, noticing the heat against my skin on this chilly morning. "What a simple pleasure," I thought as I sipped it. It tasted soothing and generated a lovely glow in my belly, which – I noticed – is looking rather flat these days. I ushered a silent thank you to God for my health, and smiled, realizing how very fortunate I am. While others are concerned about getting enough, I have to cut back, an important reminder this time of year. My mind wandered to images of family and friends, and how much I benefit from their presence in my world. I surveyed my house; I'm not wealthy, but I do have a roof over my head, a fireplace, full kitchen, and belongings others couldn't even imagine. I live in an area I love. I have my health, family, friends, and faith. What do I lack? I really do have it all.

Sitting in silence with a crumpled note on my lap and a radiance emanating from deep within, I understood this was a memory in the making and I would value it forever.

The old man hadn't left a thing but had indeed given me the greatest gift of all.

World's Weirdest Diets

════════════ ∽ ════════════

It's the most wonderful time of the year; 'tis is the time for end-of-year lists. Soon we shall (whether we want to or not) know the Top Songs/Movies/Books/News Stories of the Year. TV hosts will interview the "Most Influential Celebrities." Newsweek has gone so far as to post a compilation of lists ranging from "Top Happiest Endings of the Decade" to "Worst Predictions" (which includes "A particle accelerator will end the world"). Therefore, in honor of the list spirit, I shall now bound confidently on to the bandwagon and provide – in no particular order – a compilation of some the most bizarre diets upon which I have the misfortune to stumble. (Yes, they are all real.)

Let us commence with the COOKIE DIET. One eats one meal per day that must consist of six ounces of protein, as well as at least six of a unique type of cookie each day, for a grand total of 800 calories; about one-third the required intake to maintain a healthful body. Lose your weight and get rid of that pesky hale and hearty glow – all at once! But, mmm-mmm-mmm, sure tastes great! This proves that eating cookies to lose weight makes about as much sense as getting stabbed in the eye to forget about your earache.

After a long week, I plead guilty that a part of me welcomes the SLEEPING BEAUTY DIET. The not-so-fantasy concept is: "If you aren't awake, you aren't eating." (So, what explains the crumbs in my bed?) Followers take heavy sedation and sleep for days at a time so they won't eat and will therefore whither away. Obviously one will be thinner from this approach, but this is not much healthier than the wicked-stepmother-poisoned-apple diet that never quite caught hold.

Yes, we have no bananas. That's where they're singing in Tokyo due to a shortage of the starchy fruit brought on by the popularity of the JAPANESE MORNING-BANANA DIET. People started "going bananas" after news spread of a gentleman losing approximately 25 pounds (and gaining his fiancée) while consuming only bananas and room-temperature water every morning. His story became the first of a series of banana-diet books, selling hundreds of thousands of copies.

Part of what makes this diet so attractive is its simplicity. In addition to the Spartan breakfast, eat dinner by 8PM, be in bed by midnight, and avoid alcohol and fatty foods. One might say that this diet has a huge "appeal" and it's pretty easy to "slip up on it" (insert rimshot here...)

However, while still in the primate order, the MONKEY CHOW DIET consists of only ingesting – wait for it... can you guess? ... you got it – Monkey Chow morning, noon, and night! Honestly, no monkeying around (ah, come on, you had to expect that...).

Why its founder didn't opt for a cuisine more easily accessible – such as cat food or even fish flakes – eludes me. After all, if it's 2AM and you've got a powerful hankering for a full up platter of monkey pellets, it's not like you can scamper to the nearest convenience store and stock up. Anyway, on the positive side, the MCD does makes writing a shopping list, as well as food prep a snap. List: Monkey

Chow. Preparation: Put in mouth.

Unfortunately, this program appears to have side effects, probably due to the high amount of crude fiber in the pellets. Delicately worded, one might experience "stopped up plumbing" when visiting the restroom. (Of course, from what I know of bananas, the JAPANESE MORNING-BANANA DIET might help compensate.)

18548895R00097

Made in the USA
Charleston, SC
09 April 2013